IMMUNOLOGY AND IMMUNE SYSTEM DISORDERS

CYTOKINES AND THEIR THERAPEUTIC POTENTIAL

IMMUNOLOGY AND IMMUNE SYSTEM DISORDERS

Additional books and e-books in this series can be found on Nova's website under the Series tab.

IMMUNOLOGY AND IMMUNE SYSTEM DISORDERS

CYTOKINES AND THEIR THERAPEUTIC POTENTIAL

MANZOOR AHMAD MIR
EDITOR

nova
Medicine & Health
New York

Library of Congress Cataloging-in-Publication Data

Names: Ahmad Mir, Manzoor, PhD, Department of Bioresources, School of Biological Sciences, University of Kashmir Srinagar J&K, India, Srinagar, Jammu and Kashmir, India, editor.
Title: Cytokines and their Therapeutic Potential
Description: New York: Nova Science Publishers, [2019] | Series: Immunology and Immune System Disorders | Includes bibliographical references and index.
Identifiers: LCCN 2019957072 (print) | ISBN 9781536170177 (paperback) |
ISBN 9781536170184 (adobe pdf)

Published by Nova Science Publishers, Inc. † New York

CONTENTS

PREFACE

Immunology is a distinctive subject that rose in the mid- 20th century. The subject developed as scientists started to unravel the mysteries about the defence system against pathogens. Researchers started to understand the mechanisms employed by the innate and the adaptive immune system in defence against pathogens. During the last decade, the subject of immunology has been in sharp focus as the immunotherapies against diseases like cancer and AIDS seems last hope. Employing the body's own defence system against diseases like cancer and AIDS by activating specific cells of the immune system looks promising and therapies like CAR-T cell therapy have been approved. In the first edition of the book "Immunoglobulins, Magic Bullets and Therapeutic Antibodies" we have explained the Immunoglobulins, their genetic, production of Monoclonal antibodies, use of them in diagnostics and therapeutics and the role played by immunoglobulins in overall protection of our body.

The book is organised into four volumes. The first volume comprises of ten chapters and it describe the rise, history and scope of immunology and the building blocks of the immune system *viz.*, cells, molecules and organs of the immune system. The chapter second describes the cells of the innate and the adaptive immune system and how the granulocytes and macrophages employ defence mechanisms to protect the body against pathogenic invasions. In the chapter third of this book, we have described the organs if the immune systems and how different organs are involved in the differentiation and maturation of immune cells. The chapter has also focussed on the structure of lymph nodes and their function in concentrating the antigens. In the chapter four of this book we have described the terms like antigens, immunogens, antigenicity, immunogenicity and how immunogenicity of an antigen is affected and how antigenicity of an immunogens is related to the immune response. The innate and adaptive immune systems and the different types of cells and molecules employed by the two branches of immunity have been described in a separate chapter. The structure and biology of immunoglobulins, their types and function in antigen binding and antibody dependent cellular cytotoxicity (ADCC) have been described well in chapter six. Focus has been laid on the distinction between and antibody and an immunoglobulin. The structure and function and major histocompatibility complex (MHC) has been described well in the book. The education of cells about self and non-self during their maturation and the processing and presentation of antigens by MHC bearing cells and how MHC coordinates both humoral and cell-mediated immune responses has been explained well throughout the book. The book has explained the complement system and its components, mechanisms and functions in a separate chapter. At the end of the book, we have given an insight about the vaccines, their history, development and how they are useful and helpful in the defence against diseases. The book also discusses the immune disfunction and diseases associated with the dysregulation of immune responses.

The present book volume -3 entitles "Cytokines and their Therapeutic Potential" comprises of five chapters and it describe the Origin, production and scope of cytokines which are the glycoprotein molecules of immune system around which the field of immunology revolves. The Book on Cytokines and their Therapeutic Potential comprises of five chapters and it describe the Origin, production and scope of cytokines which are the most important molecules of immune system around which the field of functional immunology revolves. This book Describes how the immune system, responds to injuries and insults by foreign antigens (bacteria, viruses etc.) and produces cytokines, which then through various immune response mechanisms protect the body against pathogenic invasions, how these glycoproteins are involved in the differentiation and maturation of immune cells, how lymph nodes are involved in concentrating the different forms of cytokines, how immunogenicity of a cytokine is affected and how a cytokine is related to the immune response. Various types of cytokines and the organization and expression of cytokine receptors are described separately. The properties, mechanistic function and therapeutic cytokines are also discussed in separate chapters. The characteristics, production and important roles played by different cytokines in research, diagnostics and therapeutics is described separately. Lastly the role of cytokines and chemokine's in infectious diseases and their importance in the detection of various kinds of diseases like Cancer, HIV-AIDS, Tuberculosis, Malaria etc. are discussed in detail separately. The book contains a reasonable number of diagrams, flowcharts and tables. Besides this various interesting and self-explanatory illustrations are incorporated to make the book useful to the students for whom it is written. The question bank which includes long answer type, short answer type and multiple choice questions with their answers at the very end of each chapter is developed to get a full grasp of the topic.

Dr. Manzoor Ahmad Mir

ACKNOWLEDGMENTS

First, I would like to thank Almighty for giving me strength, belief and good health. It is 'HE', who is the creator of everything between Heavens and earth and beyond. May 'HE', open his clandestine treasure of knowledge upon me, 'Amen'.

I am bereft of expression that would describe my gratitude and respect to my mentors Prof Talat Ahmad, Dr. Javed N Agrewala, Prof Mohammad Afzal Zargar, Prof Raid Saleem Albaradie, and Dr. Abid Hamid Dar who stood prop all the way with zealous and enthusiastic spirit of scientific adepts. I will benefit for a long time to come from their sincerity, originality and truthfulness which has nourished my intellectual maturity. I admire and respect them all for their sincerity, dedication, devotion, amazing memory, thorough knowledge and constructive criticism

Apart from above, I am indebted to a number of people who have always been a constant source of encouragement and enthusiasm directly or indirectly, to make this book entitled "The Fundamentals of Immunology". I put on record my abysmal gratitude to all those people who lent their help in every possible way with gesture whenever and wherever the same was required by me.

I feel great happiness in expressing profound thanks and venerations to my parents who supported for touching me to new zenith in every field of life and knowledge. They have been a source of great strength throughout my life, whose tear and toil with zeal in bringing a seed of loyalty, hard work, dedication and sincerity in me warrants recognition with laud.

In addition, Miss Najmu Nisa, Research Scholar BGSBU, Mr. Aariz Manzoor Mir and Mr. Umar Mehraj, Research scholar Kashmir University, deserve a special mention. At the same time I would like to thank everybody who was important to the successful realization of this book, as well as expressing my apology that I could not mention personally one by one.

To conclude, I express my intensity of emotions towards the Prime Mover Almighty in whom I have great faith.

Dr. Manzoor Ahmad Mir

In: Cytokines and Their Therapeutic Potential ISBN: 978-1-53617-017-7
Editor: Manzoor Ahmad Mir

Chapter 1

INTRODUCTION TO CYTOKINES

Umar Mehraj, Safura Nisar, Bashir Ahmad Sheikh, Syed Suhail Hamdani, Hina Qayoom and Manzoor Ahmad Mir*

Department of Bioresources, School of Biological Sciences, University of Kashmir, Jammu and Kashmir, India

ABSTRACT

The term cytokine is a generic term for any low molecular weight soluble protein or glycoprotein (generally less than 30kD), non-immunoglobulin, released by one cell population which acts as an intercellular mediator. It includes monokines, lymphokines, interleukins, interferons and others. Cytokines are involved in the immunoregulation of both innate as well as adaptive immune responses. Interferons are cytokines prepared by cells in response to viral infection, which essentially induce a generalized antiviral state in surrounding cells. Chemokines are small, positively charged secretory proteins that have a central role in guiding the migrations of various types of white blood cells (WBCs). They bind to the surface of endothelial cells, and to negatively charged proteoglycan of the extracellular matrix in organs. By binding to G-

* Corresponding Author's Email: drmanzoor@kashmiruniversity.ac.in.

protein-linked receptors on the surface of specific blood cells, chemokines attract these cells from the bloodstream into an organ; guide them to specific locations within the organ, and then help stop migration.

Keywords: Cytokines, Interferons, interleukins, macrophages, monocytes, keratocytes, endothelial cells, chondrocytes, neutrophils, lymphocytes, hormones, stimulus, signal, lymphokines, chemokines, Monokines.

OBJECTIVES

- Brief description about cytokines.
- Different groups of cytokines.
- Functional groups of cytokines in immune system.
- Other cytokines involved in defence system.

INTRODUCTION

Cytokines are small molecules that are secreted by the cells that act as a signal between the cells, in response to a stimulus and have a variety of role owing to their ability to control immune activity. They may be described as the "hormones" of the immune system. They might have an effect on the cell that secretes them and are critical to signaling between cells, with each cytokine often inducing several different biological effects. Different cells release cytokines, as each cell type releases only certain of these molecules. Cytokines may induce growth, differentiation, chemotaxis, activation, enhanced cytotoxicity etc. However, different cytokines might have similar activities and for many cytokines, with some opposing activities to be released by a particular stimulus (Figure 1). As a result, the biological effect is a factor of the sum total of all of these activities. Cytokines can be grouped on the basis of cell populations that secrete them. Some of which are discussed as under: **Monokines** are cytokines secreted by the cells of myeloid series such as: monocytes and macrophages. **Lymphokines** are cytokines secreted primarily by lymphocytes, while some cytokines are produced by both lymphocytes and myeloid cells. **Interleukin** (IL) is a term often used to describe cytokines produced by leukocytes, although some interleukins are also produced by other cell populations. **Chemokines,** a group of small heparin-binding cytokines, directs cell migration, and may also activate cells in response to infectious agents or tissue damage. **Interferons** are cytokines produced by a variety of cells in response to much viral infections. It is important to note that the same cytokine can be made by several different cell populations. For example**,** IFNα is made by most not all nucleated cells in response to viral infection. IFNγ is produced by both T-cells as well as by NK cells. IL-1 is produced by macrophages, B cells and non-immunekeratinocytes. Many different cell types make IL-6; several others make IL-4, etc. Moreover, the same cytokine can also induce different functions in different cell types. For example, TNFα can promote the proliferation of B-cells and can also activate killing mechanism in other cell populations. IFNγ activates macrophages to kill intracellular microbes, induces B-cells to switch their antibody class to IgG and induces endothelial cells to increase expression of MHC class II molecules.

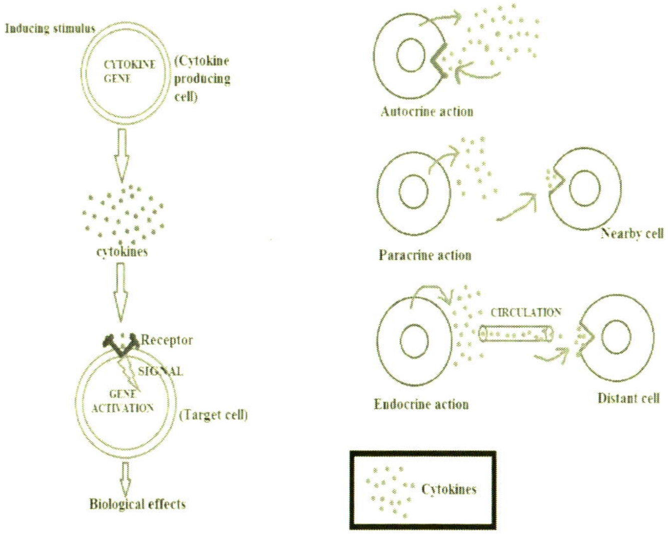

Figure 1.1. Overview of the functions of cytokines, most of which are autocrine and/or paracrine and few are endocrine in action.

Interferons

Interferons are pro-inflammatory molecules which can mediate protection against viral infection, and are thus particularly important in limiting infection during the period when specific humoral and cellular immunity is developing. They can be divided into two groups, type I IFN (IFNα and IFN-β) and type IIIFN (IFN-γ) also called immune IFN (Table 1). IFNα and IFN-β are produced by many different cells in response to viral or bacterial infections, especially by intracellular microbes. At least 12 different, highly homologous species of IFNα are produced, primarily by infected leukocytes as well as by epithelial cells and fibroblasts. In contrast, a single species of IFN-β is produced, normally by fibroblasts and epithelial cells. The pro-inflammatory cytokines IL-1 and TNFα are potent inducers of IFN-α/β secretion, as are endotoxins derived from the cell wall of Gram-negative bacteria. The receptor for both IFNα and IFN-β is the same and found on most nucleated cells. Binding of IFNα and IFN-β to this receptor inhibits protein synthesis and thus viral replication as a result of the induction of the synthesis of inhibitory proteins and of preventing mRNA translation and DNA replication. In addition, these interferons inhibit cell proliferation, increase the lytic activity of NK cells and induce increased expression of MHC class I and other components of the class I processing and presentation pathway leading to induction of antigen-specific cytolytic T-lymphocyte (CTL) responses against virally infected cells. Induction of MHC class I is also important for protection of uninfected cells from killing by NK cells. The importance of IFN-α/β in innate defense against viral infections is indicated by animal studies in which treatment of virus-infected mice with antibodies to IFN-α/β resulted in death. In contrast to the broad and rather nonspecific antiviral activity of IFN-α/β, IFNγ is primarily a cytokine of the adaptive immune system, as it is important not only for antiviral activity but also plays a major role in regulation of the development of specific immunity and in activation of cells of the immune system. Produced primarily by T_{H1} cells and NK cells, IFNγ plays a critical role in induction of T_{H1} immune responses. Early in the development of a specific immune response, IFNγ is involved in inducing differentiation of T_{H1} cells producing positive feedback for IFNγ generation and aiding CTL responses and for IgG antibody production. In addition, T_{H1} cells or CTLs responding to peptides presented in MHC molecules produce IFNγ which acts both locally and systemically to activate monocytes, and PMNs (phagocytes and macrophages) which are then better able to kill intracellular pathogens. In particular, IFNγ increases the expression of Fc receptors for IgG on PMNs as well as MHC Class II expression on a wide variety of cells. This enhances the phagocytic function of these cells as well as the antigen-presenting capabilities of professional antigen-presenting cells. IFNγ, which is crucial for macrophage function, enhances macrophage killing of intracellular bacteria and parasites probably as a result of its stimulation of their production of reactive oxygen and reactive nitrogen intermediates.

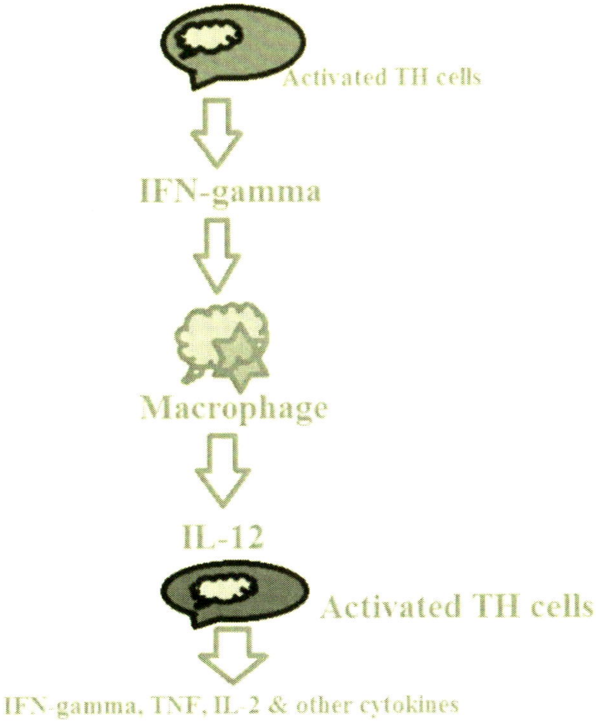

Figure 1.2. Cascade induction shown by different cytokine molecules with activated T helper cells.

Table 1. The two groups of Interferons

Group:	Type I (IFN-α/β)	Type II (IFNγ)
Chromosomal location:	9	12
Origin:	All nucleated cells, especially fibroblast, macrophages and dendritic cells.	T_{H1} cells, CD8+ cells, NK cells
Induced by:	Viruses, other cytokines, some intracellular bacteria and pathogens.	Antigen stimulated T-cells.
Functions:	Antiviral, increases MHC class-I expression, inhabits cell proliferation.	Antiviral, increases MHC class-I & class-II expression, activates macrophages.

Lymphokines

A variety of cytokines are produced by lymphocytes and lymphocyte subsets (Table 1.1), many of which are growth factors for lymphocytes and/or influence the nature of the immune response. For example, IL-2 is made by T-cells as a critical autocrine growth factor that is required for proliferation of T-cells, especially T_{H0} and T_{H1} cells and cytolytic T-lymphocyte (CTL). On activation, as a result of the interaction of their antigen receptor complexes with antigenic peptide in MHC molecules on APCs, these T-cells make IL-2 for secretion and at the same time IL-2 receptors which bind and be stimulated by the secreted IL-2. In the absence of IL-2 and/or its receptor, many antigen-specific T-cells do not express, severely affecting immune responses. IL-3 is involved in the growth and differentiation of a variety of cell types as a result of its synergistic activity with other cytokines in hematopoiesis. IL-4 is produced by both T_{H2} cells and mast cells and is a growth and differentiation factor for T_{H2} cells and B-cells. It can induce B-cell class switch to IgE antibodies. IL-4 is important in influencing the nature of the immune response, as it can induce the development of T_{H2} cells from T_{H0} cells and can inhibit the development of T_{H1} cell responses (Table 2). Thus, IL-4 is not only involved in B-cell growth, but it can also influence the B-cell and its subsequent plasma cells to produce IgE antibody. IL-5 is also produced by T_{H2} cells and mast cells and it's important for B-cell activation and in induction of B-cell class switch to IgA antibody. It also has a role in eosinophil growth and differentiation. IL-10, which is produced by T_{H2} cells and macrophages, induces B-cell activation and T_{H2} cell responses. It inhibits T_{H1} cell responses by enhancing IL-4 production and/or by suppressing macrophages activity and production of IL-12, a T_{H1}-stimulatory cytokine.

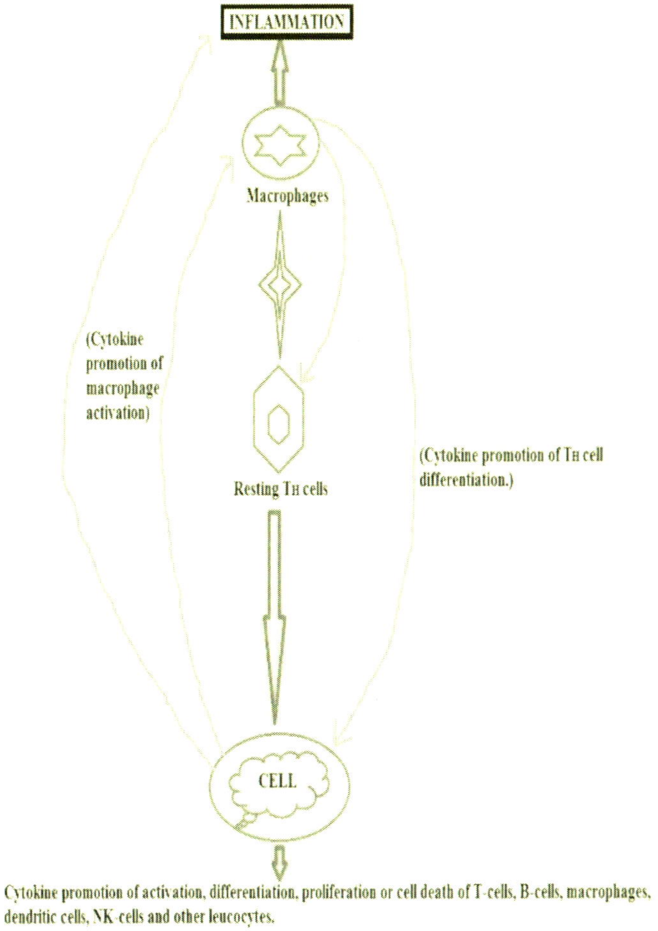

Figure 1.3. A complex network of interacting cells in the immune response which lead to the release of numerous cytokines.

Table 1.1. Different functional groups of lymphokines and Monokines

Cytokines:	Produced by:	Activity:
IL-1	Macrophages, epithelial cell	Activates vascular endothelium, tissue destruction, increased effector cell access, fever, lymphocyte activation, mobilization of neutrophils, and induction of acute phase proteins.
IL-2	T-cell	Proliferation of T-cells and NK- cells.
IL-3	T-cells, thymic cells	Proliferation and differentiation of haemopoetic cells.
IL-4	T_{H2} cells, mast cells	B-cell activation and proliferation, induces T_{H2} IgE responses and inhabits T_{H1} responses.
IL-5	T_{H2} cells, mast cells	Eosinophil growth, differentiation, B-cell activation, induces IgA responses.
IL-6	T-cells, macrophages	Lymphocyte activation, fever, induction of acute phase proteins.
IL-8	Monocytes, macrophages, fibroblasts, keratocytes	Increased tissue access for and chemotaxis of neutrophils.
IL-10	T_{H2} cells, macrophages	B-cell activation, suppression of macrophage activity, induces T_{H2} and inhabits T_{H1} responses.
IL-12	B-cells, macrophages	Induces T_{H1} and inhabits T_{H2}responses activates NK-cells.
INF-γ	T-cells, NK-cells	Macrophages and neutrophils activation induces T_{H1} and inhabits T_{H2} responses.
TNF-α	Macrophages, T-cells	Activates vascular endothelium, fever, shock, increases vascular permeability, and induces mobilization of metabolites.

Monokines

Monokines are involved in many local and systemic activities that are critical to immune defense Table 1.1. In addition, these pro-inflammatory cytokines are important mediators of inflammation. In particular, as a result of an appropriate stimulus, including ingestion of Gram-negative bacteria and subsequent activation by LPS (lipopolysaccharide), macrophages secrete IL-1, IL-6, IL-8, IL-12 and TNFα. IL-1, TNFα and IL-6 have activities which include: (1) increasing body temperature and lymphocyte activation, which decrease pathogen replication and increase specific immune responses; (2) mobilization of neutrophils for phagocytosis; (3)induction of release of acute phase proteins and thus complement activation and opsonization (Figure 1.3). IL-1 also activates vascular endothelium, in preparation for neutrophils chemotaxis and induces systemic production of IL-6. IL-8 increases access for, and chemotaxis of, neutrophils. It also activates binding by integrins, which facilitates neutrophils binding to endothelial cells and migration into tissues. Like IL-1, TNFα also activates vascular endothelium and is able to increase vascular permeability. It activates macrophages and induces their production of nitric oxide (NO). Although produced by monocytes and macrophages, TNFα is also produced by some T-cells. Finally, IL-12, which is also produced by B-cells, activates NK cells which then produce IFNγ, a cytokine important for inducing differentiation of T_{H0} cells to T_{H1} cells (Table 1.1).

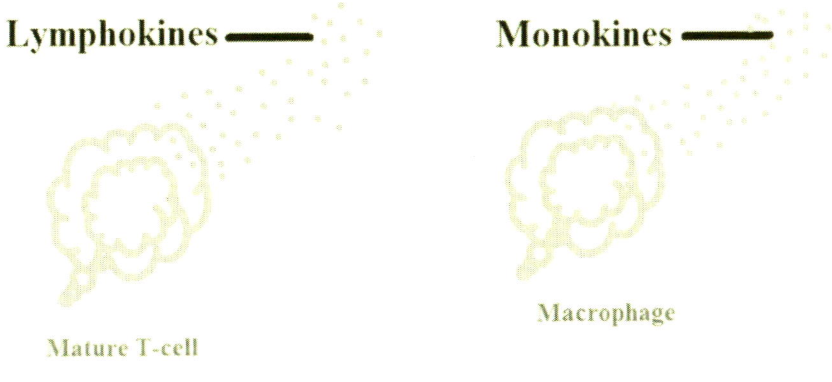

Figure 1.4. Immune responses by lymphokines and monokines.

Chemokines

This group of almost, more than 50 small, closely related cytokines (MW 8–10 kDa) are primarily involved in chemo-attraction of lymphocytes, monocytes and neutrophils (Table 1.2). These are made by monocytes/

macrophages, but also by other cells including endothelial cells, platelets, neutrophils, T-cells, keratinocytes and fibroblasts. Chemokines can be divided into four different groups based on their unique aspects of amino acid sequence, and in particular the position of conserved cysteine residues. One group has two adjacent cysteines (CC), a second has two cysteines separated by another amino acid (CXC), another has one cysteine, and the last has two cysteines separated by three other amino acids. For most of the part, CC Chemokines such as monocytes chemotactic protein (MCP-1) are chemotactic for monocytes, inducing them to migrate into tissues and become macrophages, whereas CXC Chemokines such as IL-8 are chemotactic for neutrophils inducing them to leave the blood and migrate into tissues. Some of these Chemokines are also chemotactic for T-cells.

Table 1.2. Different representative Chemokines

Class	Name	Source	Chemo-attractant for activation of
CXC (α)	IL-8 NAP-2 MIP-1b	Monocyte, Macrophage, Fibroblast, Keratocytes Platelets Monocyte, Macrophage, Endothelial cells, PMNs (neutrophils)	Naive T-cells, PMNs (neutrophils) Neutrophils CD8 T cells
CC (β)	MCP-1 Rantes	Monocyte, Macrophages, Fibroblast, Keratocytes T-cells	Memory T-cells, Monocytes Memory T_H cells
C (γ)	Lymphotactin		Lymphocytes
CX3C (δ)	Fractalkine		Lymphocytes, monocytes, NK cells

Chemokines are produced in response to an infectious process or to a physical damage and not only direct cells to the source of infection/damage, but may also enhance their ability to deal with the tissue damage. Receptors for Chemokines are all integral membrane proteins with the characteristic feature that they span the membrane seven times. These molecules are coupled to G (guanine nucleoside binding) proteins which act as the signaling moiety of the receptor. Although most of these receptors can bind more than one type of chemokine, they are usually distributed only on particular cell populations, permitting different Chemokines to have selective activity. Some Chemokines, for example IL-8 and MCP-1, have been shown to work by first binding to proteoglycan molecules on endothelial cells or on the extracellular matrix. On this solid surface they then bind blood neutrophils or monocytes, slowing their passage and directing them to migrate down a chemokine concentration gradient toward the source of the chemokine. Although the role that each plays in immune defense and pathology is still under way, it is evident that these molecules are potent agents for activating and directing effector cell populations to the site of infection and/or tissue damage as well as for controlling leukocyte migration in tissues.

Other Cytokines

Of many other cytokines which are important to immune defense, several others are particularly noteworthy (Table 1.3). A group of CSFs (colony stimulating factors), including granulocyte-monocytecolony stimulating factor (GM-CSF), Granulocyte CSF (G-CSF) and monocyte CSF (M-CSF) drive the development, differentiation and expansion of myeloid cells. GM-CSF induces expansion of myeloid progenitor cells and their commitment to the monocyte/macrophage and granulocyte lineage, after which granulocyte colony stimulating factor (G-CSF) and monocyte colony stimulating factor (M-CSF) induce specific commitment to the granulocyte or monocytes lineage respectively, and then their subsequent expansion. These factors, and especially granulocyte colony stimulating factor (G-CSF, are important clinical tools in a number of diseases, as they can be used to expand myeloid effector cell populations critical to defense against pathogens. TGF-β is produced by a variety of cells including monocytes, macrophages, T-cells and chondrocytes, and plays an important role in suppressing immune responses, as it can inhibit activation of macrophages and growth of B-cells and T-cells. TNF-β (lymphotoxin) is a molecule which is cytotoxic to a variety of cell types, including in effectual chronically infected macrophage.

Table 1.3. A list of other cytokines

Cytokine	Produced by	Activity
GM-CSF	Macrophages, T- cells	Stimulates growth, differentiation and activation of granulocytes, monocytes, macrophages.
G-CSF	Monocytes, Fibroblasts, Endothelial cells	Stimulates PMN (neutrophils) development
M-CSF	Fibroblasts	Stimulates Monocytes, Macrophages development
TGF-β	Monocytes, T-cells, Chondrocytes	Inhibits cell growth and inflammation
TNF-β (lymphotoxin)	T-cells	Cytotoxic to T, B and other cells

CONCLUSION

- Cytokines are low-molecular-weight proteins that are produced and secreted by a variety of cell types. They play major roles in the induction and regulation of the cellular interactions involving cells of the immune, inflammatory and hematopoietic systems.
- The biological activities of cytokines exhibit pleiotropy, redundancy, synergy, antagonism, and, in some instances, cascade induction.
- There are over 200 different cytokines, most of which fall into one of the following families: hematopoietins, interferons, chemokines, and tumor necrosis factors.
- Cytokines act by binding to cytokine receptors, most of which can be classified as immunoglobulin super family receptors, class I cytokine receptors, class II cytokine receptors, members of the TNF receptor family, and chemokine receptors.
- A cytokine can only act on a cell that expresses a receptor for it. The activity of particular cytokines is directed to specific cells by regulation of the cell's profile of cytokine.
- Antigen stimulation of T_H cells in the presence of certain cytokines can lead to the generation of subpopulations of helper T cells known

as T_{H1} and T_{H2}. Each subset displays characteristic and different profiles of cytokine secretion.

- The cytokine profile of T_{H1} cells supports immune responses that involve the marshalling of phagocytes, CTLs, and NK cells to eliminate intracellular pathogens. T_{H2} cells produce cytokines that support production of particular immunoglobulin isotypes and IgE-mediated responses.
- Therapies using cytokines and cytokine receptors have most clinical practice.

FREQUENTLY ASKED QUESTIONS

Q1. What are cytokines?

Answer: Cytokines are small glycoproteins produced by a number of cell types, predominantly leukocytes that regulate immunity, inflammation and hematopoiesis. They regulate a number of physiological and pathological functions including innate immunity, acquired immunity and a plethora of inflammatory responses.

Q2. What are the different types of cytokines?

Answer: According to functional classification cytokines are of two types, that enhance cellular immune responses, type 1 (TNFα, IFN-γ, etc.), and type 2 (TGF-β, IL-4, IL-10, IL-13, etc.), which favour antibody responses.

Q3. Describe the properties of cytokines?

Answer: Cytokines bind to specific receptors on the membrane of target cells, triggering signal-transduction pathways that ultimately alter gene expression in the target cells. The susceptibility of the target cell to a particular cytokine is determined by the presence of specific membrane receptors. In general, the cytokines and their receptors exhibit very high affinity for each other, with dissociation constants ranging from 10^{-10} to 10^{-}

^{12} M. Because their affinities are so high, cytokines can mediate biological effects at picomolar concentrations.

Q4. What is autocrine action?

Answer: A particular cytokine may bind to receptors on the membrane of the same cell that secreted it, exerting autocrine action.

Q5. What is paracrine action?

Answer: A particular cytokine may bind to receptors on a target cell in close proximity to the producer cell, exerting paracrine action.

Q6. What is endocrine action?

Answer: A particular cytokine may bind to target cells in distant parts of the body, exerting endocrine action.

Q7. What are the cytokines secreted by Th2 cells?

Answer: The secretion of IL-4 and IL-5 by cells of the TH2 subset induces production of IgE and supports eosinophil-mediated attack on helminths (roundworm) infections. IL-4 promotes a pattern of class switching that produces IgG that does not activate the complement pathway (IgG1 in mice, for example). IL-4 also increases the extent to which B cells switch from IgM to IgE. This effect on IgE production meshes with eosinophil differentiation and activation by IL-5, because eosinophils are richly endowed with Fc receptors, which bind IgE. Typically, roundworm infections induce TH2 responses and evoke anti-roundworm IgE antibody.

MULTIPLE CHOICE QUESTIONS

Q1. Tears contain …

A. IgA
B. IgG.
C. Lysozyme.
D. All of the above.

Q2. Opsonins include …

A. Perforin.

B. Magainins.

C. C9.

D. IFNγ.

E. C3b.

Q3. Both interleukin 1 and 2 …

A. Are produced by the same cell.

B. Require complement for their biological activity.

C. Act on T cells.

D. Trigger histamine release.

Q4. Tumor necrosis factor …

A. Decreases macrophage effector functions.

B. Increases expression of adhesion molecules on endothelial cells.

C. Decreases vascular permeability.

D. Decreases blood flow.

Q5. Cytokines that directly elevate body temperature include …

A. IL-10.

B. TGF-β

C. IL-4.

D. IL-5.

E. IL-6.

Q6. Which of the following is a known inhibitor of inflammation …?

A. TNFα.

B. Nerve growth factor.

C. Protein C.

D. Neuropeptide Y.

E. Reactive oxygen species.

Q7. Type 1 thymus-independent antigens characteristically are …

A. Small peptides.
B. Bacterial proteins.
C. Viral nucleic acids.
D. Bacterial polysaccharides.
E. Haptens.

Q8. IFNγ …

A. Is produced by all nucleated cells of the body.
B. Induces Th2 responses.
C. Can activate macrophages.
D. Was discovered because of its effect on tumors.

Q9. T cells do not …

A. Make IL-2.
B. Respond to IL-4.
C. Respond to IL-2.
D. Mediate their functions solely by cell to cell contact.

Q10. TH1 cells do not …

A. Express CD4.
B. Produce IFNγ.
C. Activate macrophages.
D. Bind soluble antigen.

Q11. Properties of antigen that may influence its role in the induction of tolerance include …

A. Its nature.
B. Its route of administration.
C. The dose of antigen.
D. Maturity of the immune system.
E. All of the above.

Q12. Molecules involved in lymphocyte activation include all of the following EXCEPT …

A. CD3.

B. CD79b.

C. CD14.

D. LCK.

E. CD28.

Q13. The process involved in allowing T cells to survive in the thymus is …

A. Positive selection.

B. Negative selection.

C. Apoptosis.

D. Necrosis.

E. Complement inactivation.

Q14. Central tolerance takes place in …

A. Lymph nodes.

B. Thymus.

C. Spleen.

D. Liver.

E. Pancreas.

Q15. The main cytokine responsible for Immunosuppressing Th1 responses are …

A. IL-1.

B. IL-2.

C. IL-4.

D. IL-10.

E. TNFα.

Answer Key

1(E), 2 (D), 3(C), 4 (B), 5 (C), 6(E), 7 (D), 8 (C), 9 (D), 10 (D), 11 (E), 12 (C), 13 (A), 14 (B), 15 (D).

Assignments

Q1. Discuss in detail about cytokines?

Q2. Explain different types of cytokines involved in immune response.

Q3. Describe different functional groups of lymphokines and monokines.

Q4. Explain chemokines and represent different class of chemokines.

Q5. What role do other cytokines play in immune defense?

References

Bloom BR, Bennett B (July 1966). "Mechanism of a reaction in vitro associated with delayed-type hypersensitivity." *Science.* 153 (3731): 80–2.

Boyle JJ (January 2005). "Macrophage activation in atherosclerosis: pathogenesis and pharmacology of plaque rupture." *Curr Vasc Pharmacol.* 3 (1): 63–8.

Candace A. Gilbert, et al. Cytokines, Obesity, and Cancer: New Insights on Mechanisms Linking Obesity to Cancer Risk and Progression. *Annu. Rev. Med.* 2013. 64:45–57.

Cannon JG (December 2000). "Inflammatory Cytokines in Nonpathological States." *News Physiol. Sci.* 15: 298–303.

Carpenter LR, Moy JN, Roebuck KA (March 2002). "Respiratory syncytial virus and TNF alpha induction of chemokine gene expression involves differential activation of Rel A and NF-kappa B1." *BMC Infect. Dis.* 2: 5.

Chen HF, Shew JY, Ho HN, Hsu WL, Yang YS (October 1999). "Expression of leukemia inhibitory factor and its receptor in preimplantation embryos." *Fertil. Steril.* 72 (4): 713–9.

Chokkalingam V, Tel J, Wimmers F, Liu X, Semenov S, Thiele J, Figdor CG, Huck WT (December 2013). "Probing cellular heterogeneity in cytokine-secreting immune cells using droplet-based microfluidics." *Lab Chip.* 13 (24): 4740–4.

Cohen S, Bigazzi PE, Yoshida T (April 1974). "Commentary. Similarities of T cell function in cell-mediated immunity and antibody production." *Cell. Immunol.* 12 (1): 150–9.

"Cytokine" in John Lackie. *A Dictionary of Biomedicine*. Oxford University Press. 2010. ISBN 9780199549351.

"Cytokine" in *Stedman's Medical Dictionary*, 28th ed. Wolters Kluwer Health, Lippincott, Williams & Wilkins (2006).

David F, Farley J, Huang H, Lavoie JP, Laverty S (April 2007). "Cytokine and chemokine gene expression of IL-1beta stimulated equine articular chondrocytes." *Vet Surg.* 36 (3): 221–7.

David JR (July 1966). "Delayed hypersensitivity in vitro: its mediation by cell-free substances formed by lymphoid cell-antigen interaction." *Proc. Natl. Acad. Sci. U.S.A.* 56 (1): 72–7.

Dimitrov, Dimiter S. (2012). "Therapeutic Proteins." *Methods in Molecular Biology.* 899. pp. 1–26.

Dinarello CA (August 2000). "Proinflammatory cytokines." *Chest.* 118 (2): 503–8.

Dowlati Y, Herrmann N, Swardfager W, Liu H, Sham L, Reim EK, Lanctôt KL (March 2010). "A meta-analysis of cytokines in major depression." *Biol. Psychiatry.* 67 (5): 446–57.

Dumonde DC, Wolstencroft RA, Panayi GS, Matthew M, Morley J, Howson WT (October 1969). ""Lymphokines": non-antibody mediators of cellular immunity generated by lymphocyte activation." *Nature.* 224 (5214): 38–42.

Gaffen SL (August 2009). "Structure and signalling in the IL-17 receptor family." *Nat. Rev. Immunol.* 9 (8): 556–67.

Giovanni Germano, et al. Cytokines as a key component of cancer-related inflammation. *Cytokine* 43 (2008) 374–379.

Haddad, E., et al. 1995. Treatment of Chediak-Higashi syndrome by allogenic bone marrow transplantation: report of 10 cases. *Blood* 11:3328.

Horst Ibelgaufts. Recombinant cytokines in *Cytokines & Cells Online Pathfinder Encyclopedia* Version 31.4 (Spring/Summer 2013 Edition).

Isaacs A, Lindenmann J (September 1957). "Virus interference. I. The interferon." *Proc. R. Soc. Lond. B Biol. Sci.* 147 (927): 258–67.

James, William; Berger, Timothy; Elston, Dirk (2005). *Andrews' Diseases of the Skin: Clinical Dermatology*. (10th ed.). Saunders.

Jump up to Said EA, Dupuy FP, Trautmann L, Zhang Y, Shi Y, El-Far M, et al. (April 2010). "Programmed death-1-induced interleukin-10 production by monocytes impairs CD4+ T cell activation during HIV infection." *Nat. Med.* 16 (4): 452–9.

Kagi, D., et al. 1994. Fas and perforin as major mechanisms of T-cell–mediated cytotoxicity. *Science* 265:528.

Key LL, Rodriguiz RM, Willi SM, Wright NM, Hatcher HC, Eyre DR, Cure JK, Griffin PP, Ries WL. (June 1995). "Long-term treatment of osteopetrosis with recombinant human interferon gamma." *N. Engl. J. Med.* 332 (24): 1594–9.

Klenerman, P., et al. 2002. Tracking T cells with tetramers: new tales from new tools. *Nature Reviews Immunology* 2:263.

Lekstrom-Himes, JA, and JI Gallin. 2000. Advances in immunology: immunodeficiency diseases caused by defects in phagocytes. *N. Engl. J. Med.* 343:1703.

Lierova A, Jelicova M, Nemcova M, et al. Cytokines and radiation-induced pulmonary injuries. *J Radiat Res.* 2018;59(6):709–753. doi:10.1093/jrr/rry067.

Locksley RM, Killeen N, Lenardo MJ (February 2001). "The TNF and TNF receptor superfamilies: integrating mammalian biology." *Cell.* 104 (4): 487–501.

Long, EO. 1999. Regulation of immune responses through inhibitory receptors. *Annu. Rev. Immunol.* 17:875–904.

Makhija R, Kingsnorth AN. (2002). "Cytokine storm in acute pancreatitis." *J Hepatobiliary Pancreat Surg.* 9 (4): 401–10.

Meager T. *The Molecular Biology of Cytokines*. New York: John Wiley & Sons; 1998.

Natarajan, K., et al. 2002. Structure and function of naturalkiller-cell receptors: multiple molecular solutions to self, nonself discrimination. *Annu. Rev. Immunol.* 20:853.

Nicolini, A et al. Cytokines in breast cancer. *Cytokine & Growth Factor Reviews* 17 (2006) 325–337.

Reche, PA (April 2019). "The tertiary structure of γc cytokines dictates receptor sharing." *Cytokine.* 116: 161–168.

Rozwarski, Denise A; Gronenborn, Angela M; (March 1994). "Structural comparisons among the short-chain helical cytokines." *Structure.* 2 (3): 159–173.

Russell, JH, and TJ Ley. 2002. Lymphocyte-mediated cytotoxicity. *Annu. Rev. Immunol.* 20:370.

Saito S (2001). "Cytokine cross-talk between mother and the embryo/placenta." *J. Reprod. Immunol.* 52 (1–2): 15–33.

Swardfager W, Lanctôt K, Rothenburg L, Wong A, Cappell J, Herrmann N (November 2010). "A meta-analysis of cytokines in Alzheimer's disease." *Biol. Psychiatry.* 68 (10): 930–41.

Tian B, Nowak DE, Brasier AR (September 2005). "A TNF-induced gene expression program under oscillatory NF-kappaB control." *BMC Genomics.* 6: 137.

Vlahopoulos SA, Cen O, Hengen N, Agan J, Moschovi M, Critselis E, Adamaki M, Bacopoulou F, Copland JA, Boldogh I, Karin M, Chrousos GP (August 2015). "Dynamic aberrant NF-κB spurs tumorigenesis: a new model encompassing the microenvironment." *Cytokine Growth Factor Rev.* 26 (4): 389–403.

Vlahopoulos S, Boldogh I, Casola A, Brasier AR (September 1999). "Nuclear factor-kappaB-dependent induction of interleukin-8 gene expression by tumor necrosis factor alpha: evidence for an antioxidant sensitive activating pathway distinct from nuclear translocation." *Blood.* 94 (6): 1878–89.

Wheelock EF (July 1965). "Interferon-Like Virus-Inhibitor Induced in Human Leukocytes by Phytohemagglutinin." *Science.* 149 (3681): 310–1.

Woodman RC, Erickson RW, Rae J, Jaffe HS, Curnutte JT (March 1992). "Prolonged recombinant interferon-gamma therapy in chronic granulomatous disease: evidence against enhanced neutrophil oxidase activity." *Blood.* 79 (6): 1558–62.

Zhang JM, An J (2007). "Cytokines, inflammation, and pain." *Int Anesthesiol Clin.* 45 (2): 27–37.

Zhu H, Wang Z, Yu J, et al. (March 2019). "Role and mechanisms of cytokines in the secondary brain injury after intracerebral hemorrhage." *Prog Neurobiol.* 178:101610.

In: Cytokines and Their Therapeutic Potential ISBN: 978-1-53617-017-7
Editor: Manzoor Ahmad Mir

Chapter 2

CYTOKINES AND THEIR TYPES

Manzoor Ahmad Mir*, Umar Mehraj, Safura Nisar, Bashir Ahmad Sheikh, Syed Suhail Hamdani and Hina Qayoom

Department of Bioresources, School of Biological Sciences,
University of Kashmir, Srinagar Jammu and Kashmir, India

ABSTRACT

Cytokines are a broad category of small proteins (~5–20 kDa) that are important in cell signaling. Their release has an effect on the behaviour of cells around them. It can be said that cytokines are involved in autocrine, paracrine and endocrine signaling as immune-modulating agents. Cytokines may include chemokines, interferons, interleukins, lymphokines, and tumor necrosis factors but generally not hormones or growth factors. Cytokines are produced by a wide range of cells, including immune cells like macrophages, B-lymphocytes, T- lymphocytes and mast cells, as well as endothelial cells, fibroblasts, and various stromal cells; a given cytokine may be produced by more than one type of the cell. They act through receptors, and are important in the immune system functioning; cytokines modulate the balance between humoral and cell-based immune

* Corresponding Author's Email: drmanzoor@kashmiruniversity.ac.in.

responses, as they regulate the maturation, growth, and responsiveness of particular cell populations. Some cytokines enhance or inhibit the action of other cytokines in complex ways. They are different from hormones, which are also important cell signaling molecules, in that hormones circulate in higher concentrations and tend to be made by specific kinds of cells. They are important in health and disease, specifically when host responses to infection, immune responses, inflammation, trauma, sepsis, cancer, and reproduction.

Keywords: macrophages, inflammation, B-lymphocytes, T-lymphocytes, interferons, chemokines, humoral immunity, fibroblasts, health, disease, autocrine, helminths, immunodeficiency, paracrine, infection, MHC-class, receptor, affinity

OBJECTIVES

- To give an outline of cytokines.
- Highlight the Insights into the discovery of cytokines.
- Discuss various properties of cytokines.
- Describe different types of cytokines.
- Understand various types of cytokine receptors.
- Discuss the T cell secreted cytokines.

INTRODUCTION

The development of an effective Immune response involves lymphoid cells, inflammatory cells, and hematopoietic cells. The complex interactions among these cells are mediated by a group of proteins collectively designated cytokines to denote their role in cell-to-cell communication. Cytokines are low-molecular weight regulatory proteins or glycoproteins secreted by white blood cells and various other cells in the body in response to a number of stimuli. These proteins assist in regulating the development of immune effector cells, and some cytokines possess direct effector functions of their own.

DISCOVERY OF CYTOKINES

Interferon-alpha (IFN-α), a type I interferon, was identified in 1957 as a protein that interfered with viral replication. The activity of interferon-gamma (IFN-γ), which is a sole member of the type II interferon class, was described in 1965; this was the first identified lymphocyte-derived mediator. Macrophage migration inhibitory factor (MIF) was identified simultaneously in 1966 by John David and Barry Bloom. In 1969 Dudley Dumonde proposed the term "lymphokine" to describe proteins secreted from lymphocytes and later, proteins derived from macrophages and monocytes in culture were called "monokines." In 1974, Stanley Cohen published an article describing the production of Macrophage migration inhibitory factor (MIF) in virus-infected allantoic membrane and kidney cells, showing its production is not limited to immune cells. This led to the proposal of term cytokine. For discovery timeline of various cytokines please see figure 1.

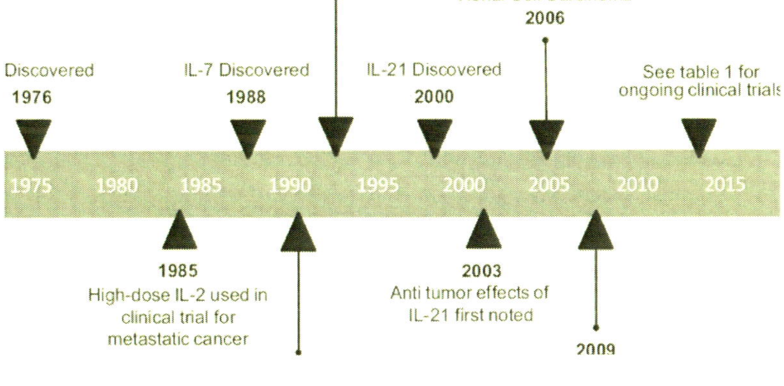

Figure 2.1. showing the timeline of discovery of various cytokines from 1976 to 2015. (Source of Image DOI: 10.1016/j.imlet.2015.11.007).

PROPERTIES OF CYTOKINES

Cytokines bind to specific receptors on the membrane of target cells, triggering signal-transduction pathways that ultimately alter gene expression in the target cells. The susceptibility of the target cell to a particular cytokine is determined by the presence of specific membrane receptors. In general, the cytokines and their receptors exhibit very high affinity for each other, with dissociation constants ranging from 10^{-10} to 10^{-12} M. Because their affinities are so high, cytokines can mediate biological effects at picomolar concentrations.

A particular cytokine may bind to receptors on the membrane of the same cell that secreted it, exerting autocrine action; it may bind to receptors on a target cell in close proximity to the producer cell, exerting paracrine action; in a few cases, it may bind to target cells in distant parts of the body, exerting endocrine action (Figure 2). Cytokines regulate the intensity and duration of the immune response by stimulating or inhibiting the activation, proliferation, and/or differentiation of various cells and by regulating the secretion of antibodies or other cytokines. The binding of a given cytokine to responsive target cells generally stimulates increased expression of cytokine receptors and secretion of other cytokines, which affect other target cells in-turn. Thus, the cytokines secreted by even a small number of lymphocytes activated by antigen can influence the activity of numerous cells involved in the immune response. For example, cytokines produced by activated T_H cells can influence the activity of B-cells, T-cells, natural killer cells, macrophages, granulocytes, and hematopoietic stem cells, thereby activating an entire network of interacting cells. Cytokines exhibit the attributes of pleiotropy, redundancy, synergy, antagonism, and cascade induction, which permit them to regulate cellular activity in a coordinated, interactive way. A given cytokine that has different biological effects on different target cells has a pleiotropic action. Two or more cytokines that mediate similar functions are said to be redundant. Redundancy makes it difficult to ascribe a particular activity to a single cytokine. Cytokine synergism occurs when the combined effect of two cytokines on cellular activity is greater than the additive effects of the individual cytokines. In some cases, cytokines exhibit antagonism, that is, the effects of one cytokine inhibitor offset the effects of another cytokine. Cascade induction occurs when the action of one cytokine on a target cell induces that cell to produce one or more other cytokines, which in turn may induce other target cells to produce other cytokines. The term *cytokine* encompasses those cytokines secreted by lymphocytes, substances formerly known as lymphokines, and those secreted by monocytes and macrophages, substances formerly known as monokines. Although these two terms continue to be used, as they are misleading because secretion of many lymphokines and monokines are not limited to lymphocytes and monocytes, but extends to a broad spectrum of cells and types. For this reason, the more inclusive term cytokine is preferred. Many cytokines are referred to as interleukins, a name indicating that they are secreted by some leukocytes and act upon other leukocytes. Interleukins 1–25 have been identified. There is a reason to support that still other cytokines will be discovered and that the interleukin group will expand further. Some cytokines are known by common names, including the interferons and tumor necrosis factors. Recently gaining prominence is yet another sub group of cytokines, the chemokines, a group of low-molecular weight cytokines that affect chemotaxis and other aspects of leukocyte behaviour. These molecules play an important role in the inflammatory response. Because cytokines share many properties with hormones and growth factors, the distinction between these three classes of mediators is often blurred. All three are secreted soluble factors that elicit their biological effects at picomolar concentrations by binding to receptors on target cells. Growth factors tend to be produced constitutively, whereas cytokines and hormones are secreted in response to discrete stimuli, and secretion is short-lived, generally ranging from a few hours to a few days.

Unlike hormones, which generally act long range in an endocrine fashion, most cytokines act over a short distance in an autocrine or paracrine fashion. In addition, most hormones are produced by specialized glands and tend to have a unique action on one or a few types of target cell. In contrast, cytokines are often produced by, and bind to, a variety of cells. The activity of cytokines was first recognized in the mid-1960s, when supernatants derived from in vitro cultures of lymphocytes were found to contain factors that could regulate proliferation, differentiation, and maturation of allergenic immune-system cells. Soon after, it was discovered that the production of these factors by cultured lymphocytes was induced by activation with antigen or with non-specific mitogens. Biochemical isolation and purification of cytokines was hampered because of their low concentration in culture supernatants and the absence of well-defined assay systems for individual cytokines. A great advance was made with the development of gene-cloning techniques during the 1970sand 1980s, which made it possible to produce pure cytokines by expressing the protein from cloned genes. The discovery of cell lines whose growth depended on the presence of a particular cytokine provided researchers with the first simple assay systems. The derivation of monoclonal antibodies specific for each of the more important cytokines has made it possible to develop rapid quantitative immunoassays for each of them.

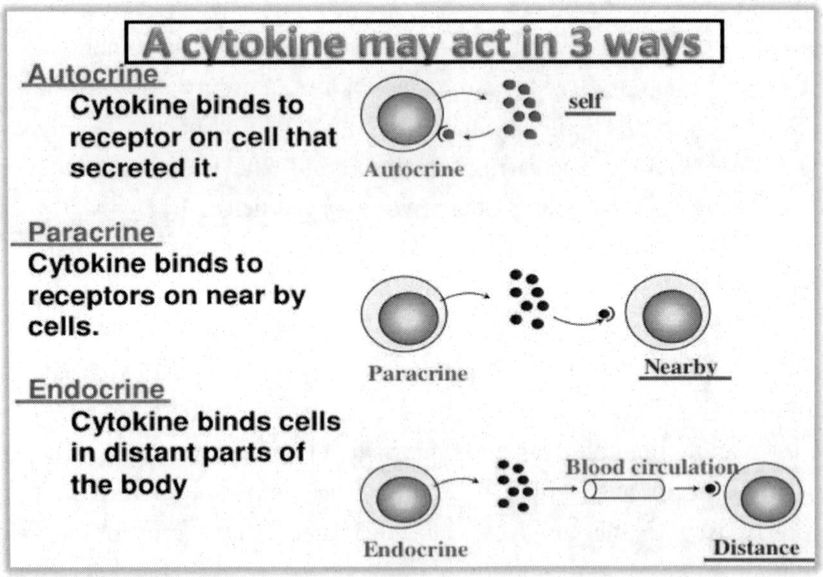

Figure 2.2. A cytokine in response to target cells.

CLASSIFICATION

1. Structural classification: Structural homogeneity has been able to partially distinguish between cytokines that do not demonstrate a considerable degree of redundancy so that they can be classified into four types:

   A. The four-α-helix bundle family: member cytokines have three-dimensional structure with four bundles of α-helices. This family, in turn, is divided into three sub-families:
      1. The IL-2 subfamily.
      2. The interferon (IFN) subfamily.
      3. The IL-10 subfamily.

The first of these three, the IL-2 subfamily, is the largest. It contains several non-immunological cytokines including erythropoietin (EPO) and thrombopoietin (TPO). Furthermore, four-α-helix bundle cytokines can be grouped into *long-chain* and *short-chain* cytokines.

   B. The IL-1 family: which primarily includes IL-1 and IL-18
   C. The IL-17 family: which has yet to be completely characterized, though member cytokines have a specific effect in promoting proliferation of T-cells that cause cytotoxic effects?
   D. The cysteine-knot cytokines: include members of the Transforming growth factor TGF-β super family, including TGF-β1, TGF-β2 and TGF-β3.

2. Functional classification: A classification that proves more useful in clinical and experimental practice outside of structural biology divides immunological cytokines into those that enhance cellular immune responses, type 1 (TNFα, IFN-γ, etc.), and type 2 (TGF-β, IL-4, IL-10, IL-13, etc.), which favour antibody responses.

A key focus of interest has been that cytokines in one of these two subsets tend to inhibit the effects of those in the other. Deregulation of this tendency is under intensive study for its possible role in the pathogenesis of autoimmune disorders. Several inflammatory cytokines are induced by oxidative stress. The fact that cytokines themselves trigger the release of other cytokines and also lead to increased oxidative stress makes them important in chronic inflammation, as well as other immune responses, such as fever and acute phase proteins of the liver (IL-1,6,12, IFN-α). Cytokines also play a role in anti-inflammatory pathways and are a possible therapeutic treatment for pathological pain from inflammation or peripheral nerve injury. There are both pro-inflammatory and anti-inflammatory cytokines that regulate this pathway.

Cytokine Receptors

To exert their biological effects, cytokines must first bind to specific receptors expressed on the membrane of responsive target cells. Because these receptors are expressed by many types of cells, the cytokines can affect a diverse array of cells. Biochemical characterization of cytokine receptors initially progressed at a very slow pace because their levels on the membrane of responsive cells are quite low. As with the cytokines themselves, cloning of the genes encoding cytokine receptors has led to rapid advances in the identification and characterization of these receptors. Cytokine receptors Fall within Five Families.

Immunoglobulin Super Family Receptors

Receptors for the various cytokines are quite diverse structurally, but almost all belong to one of five families of receptor proteins:

- Immunoglobulin super family receptors.

- Class I cytokine receptor family (also known as the hematopoietin receptor family).
- Class II cytokine receptor family (also known as the interferon receptor family).
- TNF receptor family.
- Chemokine receptor family.

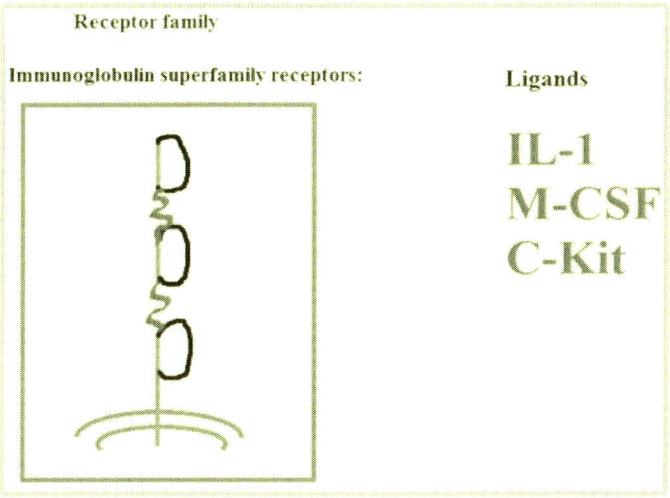

Figure 2.3. Cytokine receptors of immunoglobulin super-family.

Class I Cytokine Receptor Family (Also Known as the hematopoietin receptor Family)

Many cytokine receptors are members of the class I cytokine receptor family also called as the hematopoietin receptor family. This family was named after its first member, the hematopoietin receptor was defined. This type of receptor family has certain conserved motifs in their extracellular amino-acid domain and lacks an intrinsic protein tyrosine kinase activity. This family includes receptors for: IL2 (β-subunit), IL3, IL4, IL5, IL6, IL7, IL9, IL11, IL12, GM-CSF, Epo as well as the receptors for thrombopoietin (TPO), prolactin and growth hormone(Figure 2.2).

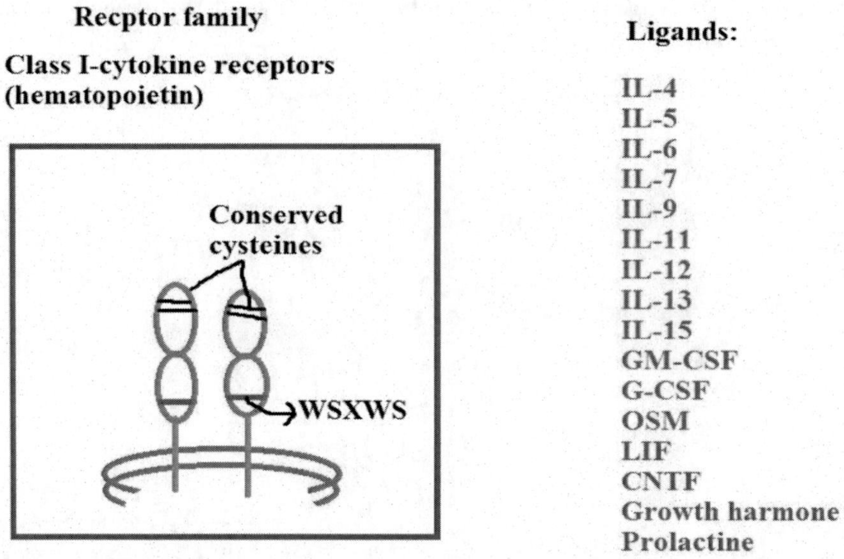

Figure 2.4. Class I Cytokine receptors (hematopoietin).

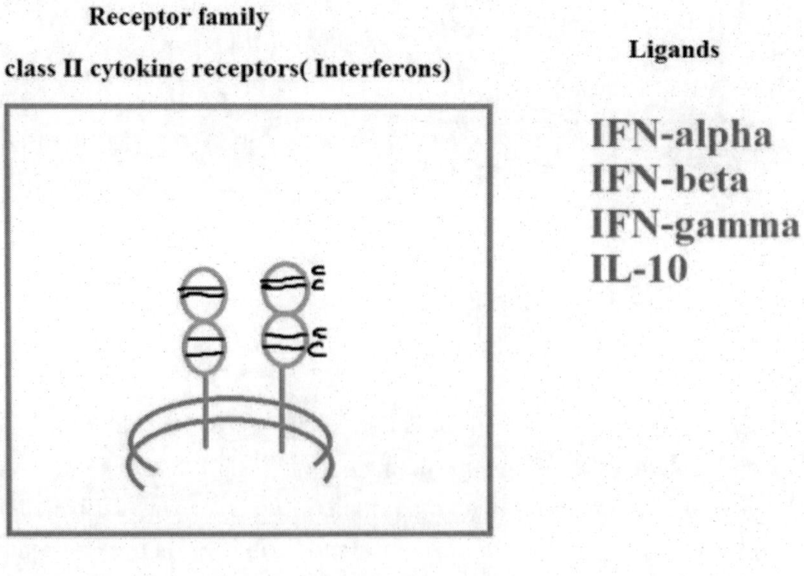

Figure 2.5. Class II cytokine receptors (Interferons).

Class II Cytokine Receptor Family (Also Known as the Interferon Receptor Family)

This type of receptor family includes a smaller number of receptors of which many are the receptors for interferons or interferon-like cytokines. Receptors included in this family are: IFN-α, IFN-β, IFNγ, IL-10, IL-22 and tissue factor (Figure 2.3). The extracellular domains of this type of receptor share structural similarities with their ligand binding domain. A number of conserved intracellular sequence motifs have been defined that function as binding sites for intracellular effector proteins JAK and STAT proteins.

TNF Receptor Family

TNF-receptor family also called as tumor necrosis receptor (TNFR) family. Its members share a cysteine-rich domain (CRD) formed of three disulphide bonds surrounding a core motif of CXXCXXC creating an elongated molecule (Figure 2.4). TNFR is associated with procaspases through adaptor proteins (FADD, TRADD, etc.) which can cleave other in-active procaspases and trigger the caspase cascade, irreversibly committing the cell to apoptosis.

Chemokine Receptor Family

This family of receptors are GPCRs with seven transmembrane structure and couple to G-protein for signal transduction (Figure 2.5). Such receptors are divided into different families like: CC chemokine receptor, CXC chemokine receptor, CX3C chemokine receptors, and XC chemokine receptor (XCR1).

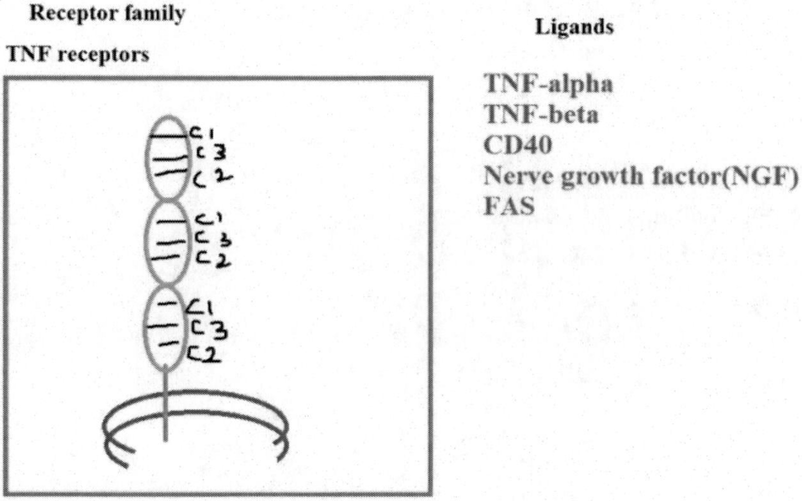

Figure 2.6. Cytokine receptors of TNF family.

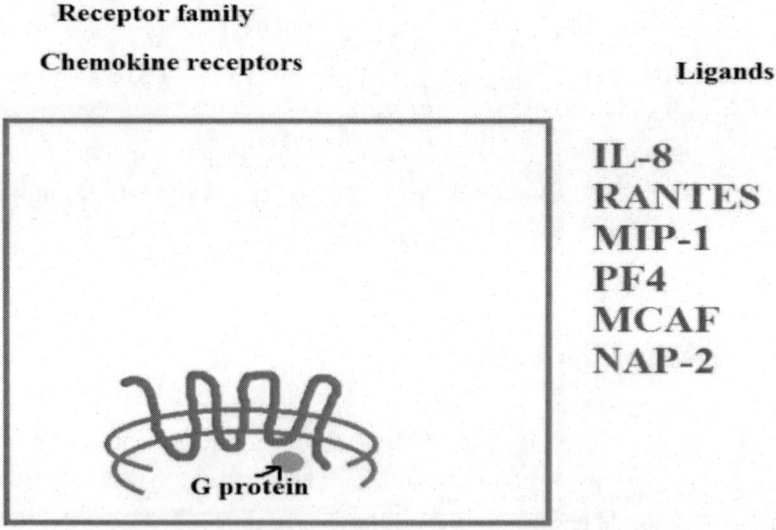

Figure 2.7. Cytokine receptors of chemokine family.

Many of the cytokine-binding receptors that function in the immune and hematopoietic systems belong to the class I cytokine receptor family. The members of this receptor family have conserved amino acid sequence motifs in the extracellular domain consisting of four positionally conserved cysteine residues (CCCC) and a conserved sequence of tryptophan serine-(any amino acid)-tryptophan-serine (WSXWS, where X is the non conserved amino acid). The receptors for all the cytokines classified as hematopoietins belong to the class I cytokine receptor family, which also is called the hematopoietin receptor family. The class II cytokine receptors possess the conserved CCCC motifs, but lack the WSXWS motif presents in class I cytokine receptors. Initially only the three interferons, α, β, and γ, were thought to be ligands for these receptors. However, recent work has shown that the IL-10 receptor is also a member of this group. Another feature common to most of the hematopoietin, class I cytokine and the class II cytokine receptor families is multiple subunits, often including one subunit that binds specific cytokine molecules and another that mediates signal transduction. However, these two functions are not always confined to one subunit or the other.

Engagement of all of the class I and class II cytokine receptors studied to date has been shown to induce tyrosine phosphorylation of the receptor through the activity of protein tyrosine kinases closely associated with the cytosolic domain of the receptors. Subfamilies of Class I Cytokine Receptors Have Signaling Subunits in Common. Several subfamilies of class I cytokine receptors have been identified, with all the receptors in a subfamily having an identical signal-transducing subunit. The sharing of signal-transducing subunits among receptors explains the redundancy and antagonism exhibited by some cytokines. Consider the GM-CSF receptor sub family, which includes the receptors for IL-3, IL-5, and GM-CSF.

Each of these cytokines binds to a unique low affinity, cytokine-specific receptor consisting of an α sub unit only. All three low-affinity subunits can associate non-covalently with a common signal-transducing β subunit. The resulting dimeric receptor not only exhibits increased affinity for the cytokine but also can transduce a signal across the membrane after binding the cytokine. Interestingly, IL-3, IL-5, and GM-CSF exhibit considerable redundancy. IL-3 and GM-CSF act upon hematopoietic stem cells and progenitor cells, activate monocytes, and induce megakaryocyte differentiation. All three of these cytokines induce eosinophil proliferation and basophile degranulation with release of histamine. Since the receptors for IL-3, IL-5, and GM-CSF share a common signal-transducing β subunit, each of these cytokines would be expected to transduce a similar activation signal, accounting for the redundancy among their biological effects. In fact, all three cytokines induce the same patterns of protein phosphorylation. Furthermore, IL-3 and GM-CSF exhibit antagonism; IL-3 binding has been shown to be inhibited by GM-CSF, and conversely, binding of GM-CSF has been shown to be inhibited by IL-3. Since the signal-transducing β subunit is shared between the receptors for these two cytokines, their antagonism is due to competition for a limited number of β subunits by the cytokine-specific α subunits of the receptors.

A similar situation is found among the IL-6 receptor subfamily, which includes the receptors for IL-6, IL-11, leukaemia inhibitory factor (LIF), oncostatin M (OSM), and ciliary neurotrophic factor (CNTF). In this case, a common signal-transducing subunit called gp130 associates with one or two different cytokine-specific subunits. LIF and OSM, which must share certain structural features, both bind to the same α subunit. As expected, the cytokines that bind to receptors in this subfamily display overlapping biological activities. IL-6, OSM, and LIF induce synthesis of acute-phase proteins by liver hepatocytes and differentiation of myeloid leukaemia cells into macrophages; IL-6, LIF, and CNTF affect neuronal development, and IL-6, IL-11, and OSM stimulate megakaryocyte maturation and platelet production. The presence of gp130 in all receptors of the IL-6subfamily explains their common signaling pathways as well as the binding competition for limited gp130 molecules that is observed among these cytokines.

A third signal-transducing subunit defines the IL-2 receptor subfamily, which includes receptors for IL-2, IL-4, IL-7, IL-9, and IL-15. The IL-2 and the IL-15receptors are heterotrimers, consisting of a cytokine-specific-α chain and two chains—β and γ—responsible for signal transduction. The IL-2 receptor γ chain functions as the signal-transducing subunit in the other receptors in this subfamily, which are all dimers. Recently, it has been shown that congenital X-linked severe combined immunodeficiency (XSCID) results from a defect in the γ -chain gene, this maps to the X chromosome (Figure 2.6). The immune-deficiencies observed in this disorder are due to the loss of all the cytokine functions mediated by the IL-2 subfamily receptors.

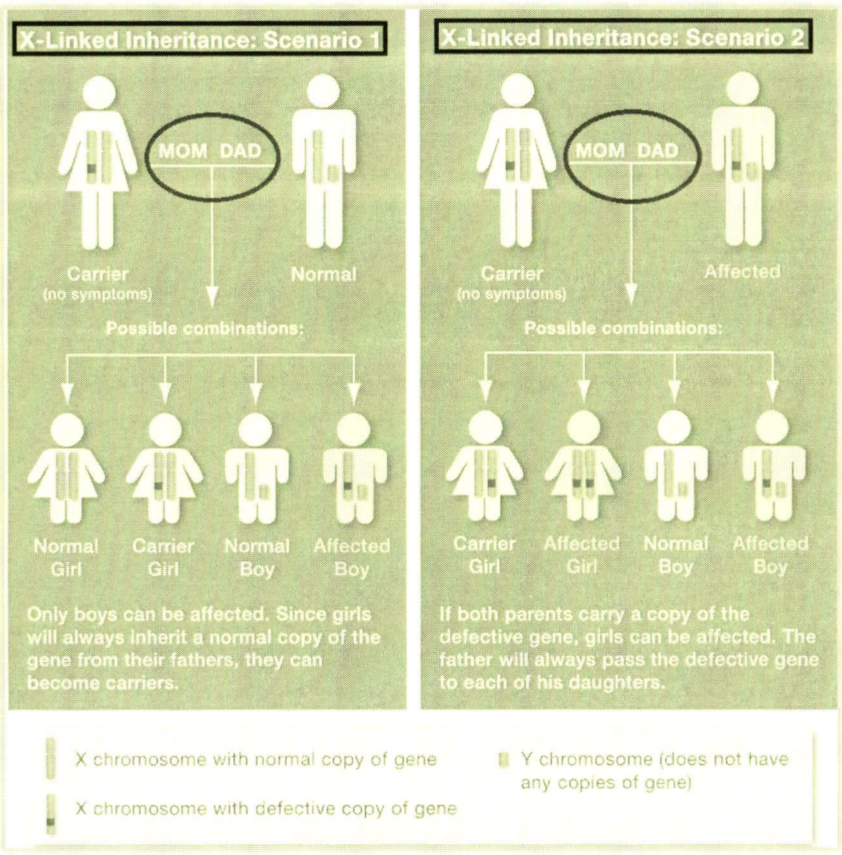

Figure 2.8. This figure depicts X-linked severe combined immunodeficiency (XSCID) syndrome among families.

The IL-2R Is One of the Most Thoroughly Studied Cytokine Receptors, because of the central role of IL-2 and its receptor in the clonal proliferation of T cells, the IL-2 receptor has received intensive study. The complete trimeric receptor comprises three distinct subunits— the α, β, and γ chains. The β and γ chains belong to the class I cytokine receptor family, containing the characteristic CCCC and WSXWS motifs, whereas the α chain has a quite different structure and is not a member of this receptor family. The IL-

2 receptor occurs in three forms that exhibit different affinities for IL-2, the low-affinity monomeric IL-2R-α, the intermediate-affinity dimeric IL-2R-βγ, and the high affinity trimeric IL-2R-αβγ. Because the α chain is expressed only by activated T-cells, it is often referred to as the TAC (T-cell activation) antigen. A monoclonal antibody, designated anti-TAC, which binds to the 55-kDa alpha chain, is often used to identify IL-2Rα on cells. Signal transduction by the IL-2 receptor requires both the β and γ chains, but only the trimeric receptor containing the α chain as well binds IL-2 with high affinity. Although the γ chain appears to be constitutively expressed on most lymphoid cells, expression of the α and β chains is more restricted and is markedly enhanced after antigen has activated resting lymphocytes. This phenomenon ensures that only antigen activated CD4+ and CD8+ T cells will express the high affinity IL-2 receptor and proliferate in response to physiologic levels of IL-2. Activated T cells express approximately 5 _ 103 high-affinity receptors and ten times as many low affinity receptors. NK cells express the β and γ subunits constitutively, accounting for their ability to bind IL-2 with an intermediate affinity and to be activated by IL-2.

Cytokine Secretion by T_{H1} and T_{H2} Subsets

The immune response to a particular pathogen must induce an appropriate set of effector functions that can eliminate the disease agent or its toxic products from the host. For example, the neutralization of a soluble bacterial toxin requires antibodies, whereas the response to an intracellular virus or to a bacterial cell requires cell-mediated cytotoxicity or delayed-type hypersensitivity. A large body of evidence implicates differences in cytokine-secretion patterns among T_H-cell subsets as determinants of the type of immune response made to a particular antigenic challenge. CD4+ T_H cells exert most of their helper functions through secreted cytokines, which either act on the cells that produce them in an autocrine fashion or modulate the responses of other cells through paracrine pathways. Although CD8+, CTLs also secrete cytokines, their array of cytokines generally are more restricted than that of CD4+ T_H cells. Two CD4+ T_H-cell subpopulations designated T_{H1} and T_{H2}, can be distinguished in-vitro by the cytokines they secrete. Both subsets secrete IL-3 and GM-CSF but differ in the other cytokines they produce. T_{H1} and T_{H2} cells are characterized by the following functional differences:

- The T_{H1} subset is responsible for many cell-mediated functions (e.g., delayed-type hypersensitivity and activation of TC cells) and for the production of opsonization-promoting IgG antibodies (i.e., antibodies that bind to the high-affinity Fc receptors of phagocytes and interact with the complement system). This subset is also associated with the promotion of excessive inflammation and tissue injury.
- The T_{H2} subset stimulates eosinophil activation and differentiation, provides help to B-cells, and promotes the production of relatively large amounts of IgM, IgE, and non-complement-activating IgG isotypes. The T_{H2} subset also supports allergic reactions.

The differences in the cytokines secreted by T_{H1} and T_{H2} cells determine the different biological functions of these two subsets. A defining cytokine of the T_{H1} subset, IFN-γ, activates macrophages, stimulating these cells to increase microbicidal activity, up-regulate the level of class-II MHC, and secrete cytokines such as IL-12, which induces T_H cells to differentiate into the T_{H1} subset. IFN-γ secretion by T_{H1} cells also induces antibody-class switching to IgG classes (such as IgG2a in the mouse) that support phagocytosis and fixation of complement. TNF-β and IFN-γ are cytokines that mediate inflammation, and it is their secretion that accounts for the association of T_{H1} cells with inflammatory phenomena such as delayed hypersensitivity. T_{H1} cells produce IL-2 and IFN-γ cytokines that promote the differentiation of fully cytotoxic T-cells from CD8+ precursors. This pattern of cytokine production makes the T_{H1} subset particularly suited to respond to viral infections and intracellular pathogens. Finally, IFN-γ inhibits the expansion of the T_{H2} population. The secretion of IL-4 and IL-5 by cells of the T_{H2} subset induces production of IgE and supports eosinophil-mediated attack on helminths (roundworm) infections. IL-4 promotes a pattern of class switching that produces IgG that does not activate the complement pathway (IgG1 in mice, for example). IL-4 also increases the extent to which B cells switch from IgM to IgE. This effect on IgE production meshes with eosinophil differentiation and activation by IL-5, because eosinophils are richly endowed with Fc receptors, which bind IgE. Typically, roundworm infections induce T_{H2} responses and evoke anti-roundworm IgE antibody. The antibody bound to the worm binds to the Fc receptors of eosinophils, thus forming an antigen-specific bridge between the worm and the eosinophils. The attack of the eosinophil on the worm is triggered by cross linking of the Fc-bound IgE. Despite these beneficial actions of IgE, it is also the Ig class responsible for allergy. Finally, IL-4 and IL-10 suppress the expansion of T_{H1} cell populations, because the T_{H1} and T_{H2} subsets were originally identified in long-term in vitro cultures of cloned T-cell lines, some researchers doubted that they represented true in-vivo subpopulations. They suggested instead that these subsets might represent different maturational stages of a single lineage. Also, the initial failure to locate either subset in humans led some to believe that T_{H1}, T_{H2}, and other subsets of T-helper cells did not occur in these species. Further research corrected these views. In many in-vivo systems, the full commitment of populations of T-cells to either the T_{H1} or T_{H2} phenotype often signals the endpoint of a chronic infection or allergy. Hence it was difficult to find clear T_{H1} or T_{H2} subsets in studies employing healthy human subjects, who would not be at this stage of a response. Experiments with transgenic mice demonstrated conclusively that T_{H1} and T_{H2} cells arise independently. Furthermore, it was possible to demonstrate T_{H1} or T_{H2} populations in T-cells isolated from humans during chronic infectious disease or chronic episodes of allergy. It is also important to emphasize that many helper T-cells do not show either a T_{H1} or a T_{H2} profile. Individual cells have shown striking heterogeneity in the T_H-cell population. One of the best described of these is the T_{H0} subset, which secretes IL-2, IL-4, IL-5, IFN-γ, and IL-10, as well as IL-3 and GM-CSF. Numerous reports of studies in both mice and humans now document that the in-vivo outcome of the immune response can be critically influenced by the relative levels of T_{H1}-like or T_{H2}-like activity (Figure 2.7). Typically, the T_{H1} profile of cytokines is higher in response to intracellular pathogens, and the T_{H2} profile is higher in allergic diseases and helminthic infections.

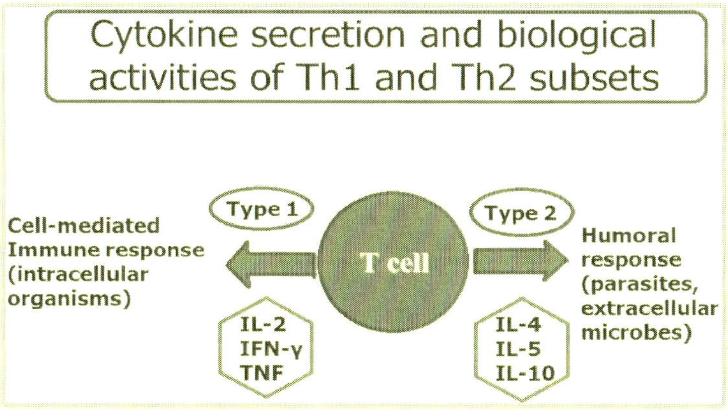

Figure 2.9. Cytokine secretion by T_{H1} and T_{H2} Subsets.

CONCLUSION

- Cytokines are small glycoproteins produced by a number of cell types, predominantly leukocytes, which regulate immunity, inflammation and hematopoiesis. They regulate a number of physiological and pathological functions including innate immunity, acquired immunity and a plethora of inflammatory responses.
- The discovery of cytokines was initiated in the 1950s, but the precise identification of their structure and function took many years.
- The original discoveries were those of IL-I, IFN and nerve growth factors (NGFs); however, these cytokines were purified and given their names years later.
- Elucidation of the precise physiological, pathological and pharmacological effects of some of the cytokines is still in progress.

- The modern techniques of molecular biology were principally responsible for their complete identification and as a consequence, several hundred cytokine proteins and genes have been identified, and the process still continues.
- Cytokines are produced from various sources during the effector phases of natural and acquired immune responses. They regulate inflammatory and other immune responses. They are also secreted during non-immune events and play a role unrelated to the immune response in many tissues. Generally, their secretion is a brief, self-limited event.
- They not only are produced by multiple diverse cell types, but also act upon many different cell types and tissues.
- Cytokines often have multiple effects on the same target cell and may induce or inhibit the synthesis and effects of other cytokines.
- A particular cytokine may bind to receptors on the membrane of the same cell that secreted it, exerting autocrine action; it may bind to receptors on a target cell in close proximity to the producer cell, exerting paracrine action; in a few cases, it may bind to target cells in distant parts of the body, exerting endocrine action.
- Cytokines regulate the intensity and duration of the immune response by stimulating or inhibiting the activation, proliferation, and/or differentiation of various cells and by regulating the secretion of antibodies or other cytokines.
- To exert their biological effects, cytokines must first bind to specific receptors expressed on the membrane of responsive target cells. Because these receptors are expressed by many types of cells, the cytokines can affect a diverse array of cells. Biochemical characterization of cytokine receptors initially progressed at a very slow pace because their level on the membrane of responsive cells is quite low.
- After binding to specific receptors on the cell surface of the target cells, cytokines produce their specific effects.

- Multiple signals regulate the expression of cytokine receptors. The target cells respond to cytokines by new mRNA and protein synthesis, which results in a specific biological response.

FREQUENTLY ASKED QUESTIONS

Q1. What are the cytokines secreted by Th1 cells?

Answer: Cytokine of the TH1 subset, IFN-γ, activates macrophages, stimulating these cells to increase microbicidal activity, up-regulate the level of class II MHC, and secrete cytokines such as IL-12, which induces TH cells to differentiate into the TH1 subset. IFN-γ secretion by TH1 cells also induces antibody-class switching to IgG classes (such as IgG2a in the mouse) that support phagocytosis and fixation of complement. TNF-β and IFN-γ are cytokines that mediate inflammation, and it is their secretion that accounts for the association of TH1 cells with inflammatory phenomena such as delayed hypersensitivity. TH1 cells produce IL-2 and IFN-γ cytokines that promote the differentiation of fully cytotoxic TC cells from CD8+ precursors. This pattern of cytokine production makes the TH1 subset particularly suited to respond to viral infections and intracellular pathogens.

Q2. What do you understand by cytokine receptors?

Answer: To exert their biological effects, cytokines must first bind to specific receptors expressed on the membrane of responsive target cells. Because these receptors are expressed by many types of cells, the cytokines can affect a diverse array of cells. Biochemical characterization of cytokine receptors initially progressed at a very slow pace because their levels on the membrane of responsive cells are quite low. As with the cytokines themselves, cloning of the genes encoding cytokine receptors has led to rapid advances in the identification and characterization of these receptors.

Q3. Describe the IL-2R?

Answer: Because of the central role of IL-2 and its receptor in the clonal proliferation of T cells, the IL-2 receptor has received intensive study. The complete trimeric receptor comprises three distinct subunits— the α, β, and γ chains. The β and γ chains belong to the class I cytokine receptor family, containing the characteristic CCCC and WSXWS motifs, whereas the α chain has a quite different structure and is not a member of this receptor family. The IL-2 receptor occurs in three forms that exhibit different affinities for IL-2: the low-affinity monomeric IL-2Rα, the intermediate-affinity dimeric IL-2Rβγ, and the high affinity trimeric IL-2Rαβγ. Because the α chain is expressed only by activated T cells, it is often referred to as the TAC (T-cell activation) antigen. A monoclonal antibody, designated anti-TAC, which binds to the 55-kDa alpha chain, is often used to identify IL-2Rα on cells. Signal transduction by the IL-2 receptor requires both the β and γ chains, but only the trimeric receptor containing the α chain as well binds IL-2 with high affinity. Although the γ chain appears to be constitutively expressed on most lymphoid cells, expression of the α and β chains is more restricted and is markedly enhanced after antigen has activated resting lymphocytes.

Q4. What are the different types of cytokine receptors?

Answer: Receptors for the various cytokines are quite diverse structurally, but almost all belong to one of five families of receptor proteins: Immunoglobulin superfamily receptors, Class I cytokine receptor family, Class II cytokine receptor family, TNF receptor family and Chemokine receptor family

Q5. What are chemokines?

Answer: The chemokines area group of low-molecular weight cytokines that affect chemotaxis and other aspects of leukocyte behaviour. These molecules play an important role in the inflammatory response.

Q6. What do you understand by pleiotropy of cytokines?

Answer: A given cytokine that has different biological effects on different target cells has a pleiotropic action.

Q7. What do you understand by redundancy of cytokines?

Answer: Two or more cytokines that mediate similar functions are said to be redundant; redundancy makes it difficult to ascribe a particular activity to a single cytokine.

Multiple Choice Questions

Q1. Chemically cytokines are

A. Proteins
B. Lipids
C. Nucleic acids
D. Glycoproteins

Q2. Which among the following is not a type 2 cytokine?

A. TNFα
B. TGF-β
C. IL-4
D. IL-10

Q3. Which among the following is not true about cytokines?

A. They exhibit pleiotropy
B. They exhibit redundancy
C. They exhibit antagonism
D. They are non-redundant

Q4. A particular cytokine may bind to receptors on the membrane of the same cell that secreted it is known as

A. Paracrine action
B. Autocrine action
C. Endocrine action
D. Cascade induction

Q5. A particular cytokine may bind to receptors on a target cell in close proximity to the producer cell is known as

A. Autocrine action
B. Paracrine action
C. Cascade induction
D. Pleiotropy

Q6. A particular cytokine may bind to target cells in distant parts of the body, exerting

A. Paracrine action
B. Autocrine action
C. Endocrine action
D. Cascade induction

Q7. What among the following are cytokines secreted by Th2 cells?

A. IL-4
B. IL-1
C. IL-2
D. IL10

Q8. What among the following are cytokines secreted by Th1 cells?

A. IFN-γ
B. IL-1
C. IL-4
D. IL-5

Q9. Which among the following is not the component of IL-2-R?

A. α chain

B. β chain

C. γ chain

D. κ peptide

Q10. Which among the following statements is not true about chemokines?

A. Affect chemotaxis

B. Affects aspects of leukocyte behavior

C. Role in the inflammatory response

D. Doesn't affect chemotaxis

Q11. Which among the following antibody is responsible for allergic reactions?

A. IgA

B. IgG

C. IgE

D. IgM

Q12. A monoclonal antibody, designated anti-TAC, which binds to the peptide of IL-2R chain, is often used to identify

A. IL-2Rα

B. IL-2Rβ

C. IL-2Rγ

D. IL-2Rβγ

Q13. What is the number of cytokine receptor families?

A. Three

B. Four

C. Five

D. Six

Q14. Which among the following is NOT a cytokine receptor family?

A. Class I cytokine receptor family
B. Class II cytokine receptor family
C. Class III receptor family
D. Chemokine receptor family

Q15. The activity of cytokines was first recognized in the

A. Mid 1950s
B. Mid- 1960s
C. Mid- 1970s
D. Mid- 1980s

Answer Key

1(D) 2(A) 3(D) 4(B) 5(B) 6(C) 7(A) 8(A) 9(D) 10(D) 11(C) 12(A) 13(C) 14(C) 15(B).

Assignments

Q1. Discuss in detail the properties of cytokines?
Q2. Describe the cytokine receptor families?
Q3. What are the different types of classifications of cytokines?
Q4. Discuss in detail the IL-2R?
Q5. Discuss synergism of cytokines.

References

Abbas, A., K. M. Murphy, and A. Sher. 1996. Functional diversity of helper T lymphocytes. *Nature* 383:787.

Alcami, A., and U. H. Koszinowski. 2000. Viral mechanisms of immune evasion. *Immunol. Today* 9:447–455.

Anne Masi, Nicholas Glozier, Russell Dale, Adam J. *Guastella Neurosci* Bull. 2017 Apr; 33(2): 194–204.

Bach, E. A., M. Aguet, and R. D. Schreiber. 1998. The IFN-_ receptor: a paradigm for cytokine receptor signaling. *Ann. Rev. Immunol.* 15:563.

Burska A, Boissinot M, Ponchel F. Cytokines as biomarkers in rheumatoid arthritis. *Mediators Inflamm.* 2014;2014:545493. doi:10.1155/2014/545493.

Carpenter LR, Moy JN, Roebuck KA (March 2002). "Respiratory syncytial virus and TNF alpha induction of chemokine gene expression involves differential activation of Rel A and NF-kappa B1". *BMC Infect. Dis.* 2: 5.

Chokkalingam V, Tel J, Wimmers F, Liu X, Semenov S, Thiele J, Figdor CG, Huck WT (December 2013). "Probing cellular heterogeneity in cytokine-secreting immune cells using droplet-based microfluidics." *Lab Chip.* 13 (24): 4740–4.

David F, Farley J, Huang H, Lavoie JP, Laverty S (April 2007). "Cytokine and chemokine gene expression of IL-1beta stimulated equine articular chondrocytes." *Vet Surg.* 36 (3): 221–7.

Darnell, J. E. Jr. 1997. STATs and gene regulation. *Science* 5332:1630–1635.

Fitzgerald, K. A., et al. 2001. *The Cytokine Facts Book,* second edition. Academic Press.

Flynn, J. L., and J. Chan. 2001. Immunology of tuberculosis. *Annu. Rev. Immunol.* 19:93–129.

Gadina, M., et al. 2001. Signaling by type I and II cytokine receptors: ten years after. *Curr. Opin. Immunol.* 3:363–373.

Gaffen SL (August 2009). "Structure and signalling in the IL-17 receptor family". *Nat. Rev. Immunol.* 9 (8): 556–67.

Jaeckel, E., et al. 2001. Treatment of acute hepatitis C with interferon _-2b. *N. Engl. J. Med.* 345:1452–1457.

Jump up to Said EA, Dupuy FP, Trautmann L, Zhang Y, Shi Y, El-Far M, et al. (April 2010). "Programmed death-1-induced interleukin-10 production by monocytes impairs CD4+ T cell activation during HIV infection". *Nat. Med.* 16 (4): 452–9.

Meager T. *The Molecular Biology of Cytokines*. New York: John Wiley & Sons; 1998.

Morel PA, Lee REC, Faeder JR. Demystifying the cytokine network: Mathematical models point the way. *Cytokine*. 2017;98:115–123.

Mossman, T. R., H. Cherwinski, M. W. Bond, M. A. Gledlin, and R. L. Coffman. 1986. Two types of murine helper T cell clone. I. Definition according to profiles of lymphokine activities and secreted proteins. *J. Immunology* 136:2348.

Nijaguna MB, Patil V, Hegde AS, et al. An Eighteen Serum Cytokine Signature for Discriminating Glioma from Normal Healthy Individuals. *PLoS One*. 2015;10(9):e0137524. Published 2015 Sep 21.

Pulliam SR, Uzhachenko RV, Adunyah SE, Shanker A. Common gamma chain cytokines in combinatorial immune strategies against cancer. *Immunol Lett*. 2016; 169:61–72.

Reche, PA (April 2019). "The tertiary structure of γc cytokines dictates receptor sharing." *Cytokine*. 116: 161–168.

Rengarajan, J., S. J. Szabo, and L. H. Glimcher. 2000. Transcriptional regulation of ThH1/ThH2 polarization. *Immunol. Today* 10:479–483.

Rozwarski, Denise A; Gronenborn, Angela M; (March 1994). "Structural comparisons among the short-chain helical cytokines." *Structure*. 2 (3): 159–173.

Stenken JA, Poschenrieder AJ. Bioanalytical chemistry of cytokines--a review. *Anal Chim Acta*. 2015;853:95–115.

Szabo, S. J. et al. 2000. A novel transcription factor, T-bet, directs TH1 lineage commitment. *Cell* 100:655–669.

Tian B, Nowak DE, Brasier AR (September 2005). "A TNF-induced gene expression program under oscillatory NF-kappaB control". *BMC Genomics*. 6: 137.

Vlahopoulos S, Boldogh I, Casola A, Brasier AR (September 1999). "Nuclear factor-kappaB-dependent induction of interleukin-8 gene expression by tumor necrosis factor alpha: evidence for an antioxidant sensitive activating pathway distinct from nuclear translocation." *Blood.* 94 (6): 1878–89.

Walter, M. R., et al. 1995. Crystal structure of a complex between interferon-_ and its soluble high-affinity receptor. *Nature* 376: 230.

Wojdasiewicz P, Poniatowski ŁA, Szukiewicz D. The role of inflammatory and anti-inflammatory cytokines in the pathogenesis of osteoarthritis. *Mediators Inflamm.* 2014;2014:561459.

Zhang JM, An J (2007). "Cytokines, inflammation, and pain". *Int Anesthesiol Clin.* 45 (2): 27–37.

In: Cytokines and Their Therapeutic Potential ISBN: 978-1-53617-017-7
Editor: Manzoor Ahmad Mir

Chapter 3

PROPERTIES AND FUNCTIONS OF CYTOKINES

Umar Mehraj, Safura Nisar, Bashir Ahmad Sheikh, Syed Suhail Hamdani, Hina Qayoom and Manzoor Ahmad Mir*

Department of Bioresources, School of Biological Sciences, University of Kashmir, Srinagar Jammu and Kashmir, India

ABSTRACT

Cytokines are small glycoproteins produced by a number of cell types, predominantly leukocytes, which regulate immunity, inflammation and hematopoiesis. They regulate a number of physiological and pathological functions including innate immunity, acquired immunity and a plethora of inflammatory responses. The discovery of cytokines was initiated in the 1950s, but the precise identification of their structure and function took many years. The original discoveries were those of IL-I, IFN and nerve growth factors (NGFs), however, these cytokines were purified and given their names years later. Elucidation of the precise physiological, pathological and pharmacological effects of some of the cytokines is still

* Corresponding Author's Email: drmanzoor@kashmiruniversity.ac.in.

in progress. The modern techniques of molecular biology were principally responsible for their complete identification and as a consequence, several hundred cytokine proteins and genes have been identified, and the process still continues.

Keywords: cytotoxicity, cytokines, allogenic, purification, differentiation, tyrosine kinase, super family, pro-inflammatory, adipogenesis, osteoclastogenesis, receptors, natural killer cells, JAKs, STAT, transcription factors.

OBJECTIVES

- To give an outline of the properties of cytokines.
- Describe the mechanism of cytokine functioning.
- Discuss different functions of cytokines.
- Discuss various types of cytokines and their mode of action.
- To discuss prominent Interleukins types in relation to diseases.

INTRODUCTION

Cytokines are produced from various sources during the effector phases of natural and acquired immune responses and regulate immune and inflammatory responses. They are also secreted during non-immune events and play a role unrelated to the immune response in many tissues. Generally, their secretion is a brief, self-limited event. They not only are produced by multiple diverse cell types, but also act upon many different cell types and tissues (Figure 3.1). Cytokines often have multiple effects on the same target cell and may induce or inhibit the synthesis and effects of other cytokines. After binding to specific receptors on the cell surface of the target cells, cytokines produce their specific effects. Multiple signals regulate the expression of cytokine receptors. The target cells respond to cytokines by new mRNA and protein synthesis, which results in a specific biological response.

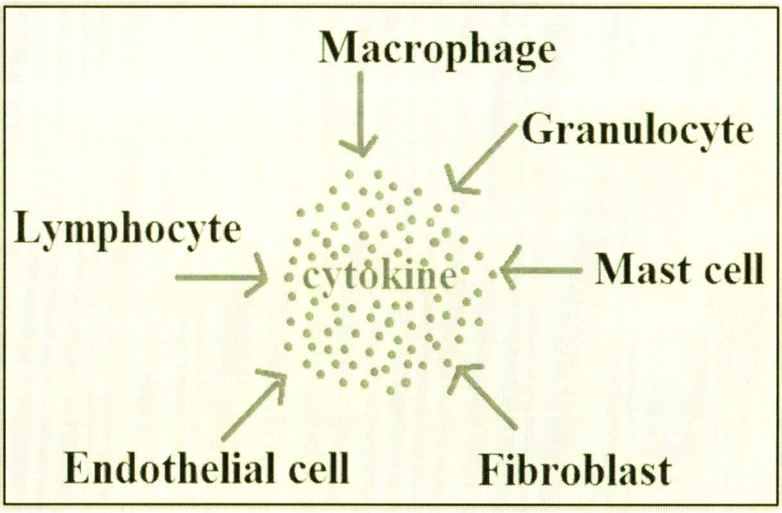

Figure 3.1. Cytokine production by different cell types.

Properties of Cytokines

The activity of cytokines was first recognized in the mid- 1960s, when supernatants derived from in vitro cultures of lymphocytes were found to contain factors that could regulate proliferation, differentiation, and maturation of allogeneic immune-system cells. Soon after, it was discovered that production of these factors by cultured lymphocytes was induced by activation with antigen or with non-specific mitogens. Biochemical isolation and purification of cytokines was hampered because of their low concentration in culture supernatants and the absence of well-defined assay systems for individual cytokines. A great advance was made with the development of gene-cloning techniques during the 1970s and 1980s, which made it possible to produce pure cytokines by expressing the protein from cloned genes. The discovery of cell lines whose growth depended on the presence of a particular cytokine provided researchers with the first simple assay systems. The derivation of monoclonal antibodies specific for each of the more important cytokines has made it possible to develop rapid quantitative immunoassays for each of them. The term *cytokine* encompasses those cytokines secreted by lymphocytes, substances formerly known as *lymphokines,* and those secreted by monocytes and macrophages, substances formerly known as *monokines.* Although these other two terms continue to be used, they are misleading because secretion of many lymphokines and monokines is not limited to lymphocytes and monocytes as these terms imply, but extends to a broad spectrum of cells and types. For this reason, the more inclusive term *cytokine* is preferred. Many cytokines are referred to as *interleukins,* a name indicating that they are secreted by some leukocytes and act upon other leukocytes. Interleukins 1–25 have been identified. There is reason to suppose that still other cytokines will be discovered and that the interleukin group will expand further. Some cytokines are known by common names, including the interferons and tumor necrosis factors. Recently gaining prominence is yet another subgroup of cytokines, the *chemokines*, a group of low-molecular weight cytokines that affect chemotaxis and other aspects of leukocyte behaviour. These molecules play an important role in the inflammatory response. Because cytokines share many properties with hormones and growth factors, the distinction between these three classes of mediators is often blurred. All three are secreted soluble factors that elicit their biological effects at picomolar concentrations by binding to receptors on target cells. Growth factors tend to be produced constitutively, whereas cytokines and hormones are secreted in response to discrete stimuli, and secretion is short-lived, generally ranging from a few hours to a few days. Unlike hormones, which generally act long range in an endocrine fashion, most cytokines act over a short distance in an autocrine or paracrine fashion. In addition, most hormones are produced by specialized glands and tend to have a unique action on one or a few types of target cell. In contrast, cytokines are often produced by, and bind to, a variety of cells.

Cytokines bind to specific receptors on the membrane of target cells, triggering signal-transduction pathways that ultimately alter gene expression in the target cells (Figure 3.2). The susceptibility of the target cell to a particular cytokine is determined by the presence of specific membrane receptors. In general, the cytokines and their receptors exhibit very high affinity for each other, with dissociation constants ranging from 10^{-10} to 10^{-12} M, because their affinities are so high, cytokines can mediate biological effects at picomolar concentrations.

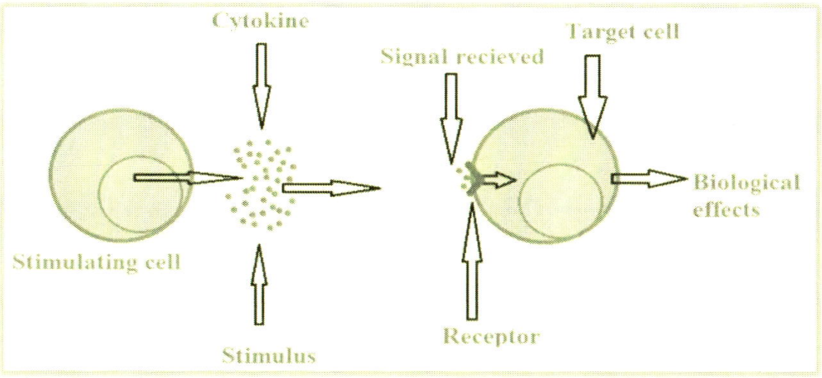

Figure 3.2. How cytokines bind to the target cells and develop biological effects.

A particular cytokine may bind to receptors on the membrane of the same cell that secreted it, exerting *autocrine* action; it may bind to receptors on a target cell in close proximity to the producer cell, exerting *paracrine* action and in a few cases, it may bind to target cells in distant parts of the body, exerting *endocrine* action. Cytokines regulate the intensity and duration of the immune response by stimulating or inhibiting the activation, proliferation, and/ or differentiation of various cells and by regulating the secretion of antibodies or other cytokines. The binding of a given cytokine to responsive target cells generally stimulates increased expression of cytokine receptors and secretion of other cytokines, which affect other target cells in turn. Thus, the cytokines secreted by even a small number of lymphocytes activated by antigen can influence the activity of numerous cells involved in the immune response. For example, cytokines produced by activated T_H cells can influence the activity of B-cells, T-cells, natural killer cells, macrophages, granulocytes, and hematopoietic stem cells, thereby activating an entire network of interacting cells. Cytokines exhibit the attributes of pleiotropy, redundancy, synergy, antagonism, and cascade induction, which permit them to regulate cellular activity in a coordinated, interactive way. A given cytokine that has different biological effects on different target cells has a pleiotropic action. Two or more cytokines that mediate similar functions are said to be redundant, redundancy makes it difficult to ascribe a particular activity to a single cytokine. Cytokine synergism occurs when the combined effect of two cytokines on cellular activity is greater than the additive effects of the individual cytokines. In some cases, cytokines exhibit antagonism, that is, the effects of one cytokine inhibit or offset the effects of another cytokine. Cascade induction occurs when the action of one cytokine on a target cell induces that cell to produce one or more other cytokines, which in turn may induce other target cells to produce other cytokines.

Functions of Cytokines

Engaged Cytokine Receptors activate Signaling Pathways: While some important cytokine receptors lie outside the class I and class II families, the majority are included within these two families. As mentioned previously, class I and class II cytokine receptors lack signaling motifs (e.g., intrinsic tyrosine kinase domains). Early observations demonstrated that one of the first events after the interaction of a cytokine with one of these receptors is a series of protein tyrosine phosphorylation. While these results were initially puzzling, they were explained when a unifying model emerged from studies of the molecular events triggered by binding of interferon gamma (IFN-γ) to its receptor, a member of the class II family. IFN-γ was originally discovered because of its ability to induce cells to block or inhibit the replication of a wide variety of viruses. Antiviral activity is a property it shares with IFN-α and IFN-β. However, unlike these other interferons, IFN-γ plays a central role in many immune regulatory processes, including the regulation of mononuclear phagocytes, B-cell switching to certain IgG classes, and the support or inhibition of the development of T_H-cell subsets. The discovery of the major signaling pathway invoked by interaction of IFN-γ with its receptor led to the realization that signal transduction through most, if not all, class I and class II cytokine receptors involves the following steps, which are the basis of a unifying signaling model:

- *The cytokine receptor is composed of separate subunits,* an α chain required for cytokine binding and for signal transduction and a β chain necessary for signaling but with only a minor role in binding.
- *Different inactive protein tyrosine kinases are associated with different subunits of the receptor.* The α chain of their receptor is associated with a novel family of protein tyrosine kinases, the Janus kinase (JAK) family. The association of the JAK and the receptor subunit occurs spontaneously and does not require the binding of cytokine. However, in the absence of cytokine, JAKs lack protein tyrosine kinase activity.
- *Cytokine binding induces the association of the two separate cytokine receptor subunits and activation of the receptor-associated JAKs.* The ability of IFN-γ, which binds to a class II cytokine receptor, to bring about the association of the ligand-binding chains of its receptor, has been directly demonstrated by x-ray crystallographic studies.
- *Activated JAKs create docking sites for the STAT transcription factors by phosphorylation of specific tyrosine residues on cytokine receptor subunits.* Once receptor associated JAKs are activated, they phosphorylate specific tyrosines in the receptor subunits of the complex. Members of a family of transcription factors known as *STATs (signal transducers and activators of transcription)* bind to these phosphorylated tyrosine residues. Specific STATs play essential roles in the signaling pathways of a wide variety of cytokines. The binding of STATs to receptor subunits is mediated by the joining of the SH2 domain on the STAT with the docking site created by the JAK-mediated phosphorylation of a particular tyrosine on receptor subunits.
- *After undergoing JAK-mediated phosphorylation, STAT transcription factors translocate from receptor docking sites at the membrane to the nucleus, where they initiate the transcription of*

> *specific genes.* While docked to receptor subunits, STATs undergo JAK-catalyzed phosphorylation of a key tyrosine. This is followed by the dissociation of the STATs from the receptor subunits and their dimerization. The STAT dimers then translocate into the nucleus and induce the expression of genes containing appropriate regulatory sequences in their promoter regions.

In addition to IFN-γ, a number of other class I and class II ligands have been shown to cause dimerization of their receptors. An important element of cytokine specificity derives from the exquisite specificity of the match between cytokines and their receptors. Another aspect of cytokine specificity is that each particular cytokine (or group of redundant cytokines) induces transcription of a specific subset of genes in a given cell type, the resulting gene products then mediate the various effects typical of that cytokine. The specificity of cytokine effects is then traceable to three factors. First, particular cytokine receptors start particular JAK-STAT pathways. Second, the transcriptional activity of activated STATs is specific because a particular STAT homodimer or heterodimer will only recognize certain sequence motifs and thus can interact only with the promoters of certain genes. Third, only those target genes whose expression is permitted by a particular cell type can be activated within that variety of cell. That is, in any given cell type only a subset of the potential target genes of a particular STAT may be permitted expression. For example, IL-4 induces one set of genes in T-cells, another in B-cells, and a third in eosinophils.

Examples of Some Cytokines

Interleukin-1

Interleukin-1was originally discovered as a factor that induced fever, caused damage to joints and regulated bone marrow cells and lymphocytes, it was given several different names by various investigators. Later, the presence of two distinct proteins, IL-1α and IL-1β, was confirmed, which belong to a family of cytokines, theIL-1 super family. Ten ligands of IL-1 have been identified, termed IL-1F1 toIL-1F10. With the exception of IL-1F4, all of their genes map to the region of chromosome 2. IL-1 plays an important role in both innate and adaptive immunity and is a crucial mediator of the host inflammatory response in natural immunity. The major cell source of IL-1 is the activated mononuclear phagocyte. Other sources include dendritic cells, epithelial cells, endothelial cells, B-cells, astrocytes, fibroblasts and large granular lymphocytes (LGL). Endotoxins, macrophage derived cytokines such as TNF or IL-1 itself, and contact with CD4+ cells trigger IL-1 production. IL-1 can be found in circulation following Gram-negative bacteria sepsis. It produces the acute-phase response in response to infection. IL-1 induces fever as a result of bacterial and viral infections. It suppresses the appetite and induces muscle proteolysis, which may cause severe muscle "wasting" in patients with chronic infection. IL-1β causes the destruction of β cells leading to type-I diabetes mellitus. It inhibits the function and promotes the apoptosis of pancreatic β cells.

Activation of T-helper cells, resulting in IL-2 secretion, and B-cell activation are mediated by IL-1. It is a stimulator of fibroblast proliferation, which causes wound healing. Autoimmune diseases exhibit increased IL-1 concentrations. It suppresses further IL-1 production via an increase in the synthesis of PGE2. IL-1s exert their effects via specific cell surface receptors that include a family of about nine members characterized as IL-1R1 to IL-1R9. All family members with the exception of IL-1R2 have an intracellular TLR domain. Each type of receptor in the family has some common and some unique features.

Interleukin-2

IL-2, a single polypeptide chain of 133 amino acid residues, is produced by immune regulatory cells that are principally T cells. When a helper T cell binds to an APC using CD28 and B7, CD4+ cells produce IL-2. IL-2 supports the proliferation and differentiation of any cell that has high-affinity IL-2 receptors. It is necessary for the activation of T cells. Resting T lymphocytes (un-stimulated) belonging to either theCD4+ or the CD8+ subsets possess few high-affinity IL-2 receptors, but following stimulation with specific antigen, there is a substantial increase in their numbers. The binding of IL-2 with its receptors on T cells induces their proliferation and differentiation. IL-2 is the major growth factor for T lymphocytes, and the binding of IL-2 to its specific receptors on T_H cells stimulates the proliferation of these cells and the release of a number of cytokines from these cells. IL-2 is required for the generation of CD8+ cytolytic T-cells, which are important in antiviral responses.

IL-2 increases the effector function of NK-cells. When peripheral blood lymphocytes are treated with IL-2 for 48–72 h, lymphokine-activated killer (LAK) cells are generated, which can kill a much wider range of targets including the tumor cells. IL-2 enhances the ability of the immune system to kill tumor cells and may also interfere with the blood flow to the tumours. It not only induces lymphoid growth but also maintains peripheral tolerance by generation of regulatory T-cells. IL-2 knockout mice produce a wide range of auto antibodies and many die of autoimmune haemolytic anaemia, which suggests that it plays a role in immune tolerance. IL-4 is a pleiotropic cytokine produced by T_{H2} cells, mast cells and NK-cells. Other specialized subsets of T-cells, basophils and eosinophils also produce IL-4. It regulates the differentiation of antigen-activated naive T-cells. These cells then develop to produce IL-4 and a number of other T_{H2}-type cytokines including IL-5, IL-10 andIL-13. IL-4 suppresses the production of T_{H1} cells. It is required for the production of IgE and is the principal cytokine that causes isotype switching of B-cells from IgG expression to IgE and IgG4. As a consequence, it regulates allergic disease. IL-4 leads to a protective immunity against helminths and other extracellular parasites. The expression of MHC class II molecules on B-cells and the expression of IL-4 receptors are up regulated by IL-4. In combination with TNF, IL-4 increases the expression of VCAM-1 and decreases the expression of E-selectin, which results in eosinophil recruitment in lung inflammation. IL-4 mediates its effects via specific IL-4 receptors that are expressed on a number of tissues including hematopoietic cells, endothelium, hepatocytes, epithelial cells, fibroblasts, neurons and muscles.

Interleukin-2 and AIDS

HIV is a retrovirus that infects CD4+ cells. After HIV becomes integrated into the genome of the CD4+ cells, activation of these cells results in the replication of virus, which causes lysis of the host cells. Patients infected with HIV, and with AIDS, generally have reduced numbers of helper T-cells and the CD4:CD8 ratio may be as low as 0.5:1 instead of the normal 2:1. As a consequence, very little IL-2 is available to support the growth and proliferation of CD4+ cells despite the presence of effector cells, B-cells and cytolytic T-cells. Proleukin has not been approved for the treatment of HIV, however, studies show that proleukin in combination with antiretroviral therapy significantly increases the number of CD4+ cells. Low-frequency doses of subcutaneous proleukin at maintained intervals increased CD4+ cell levels. The CD4 count increased from 520cells/_l to 1005 cells/_l, and the mean of CD4+ cells present from 27 to 38%. The overall effects of proleukin administration in combination with other anti-HIV drugs are being studied to determine the regulation of immune response as well as a delay in the progression of HIV disease.

Interleukin-5

IL-5 is secreted predominantly by T_{H2} lymphocytes. However, it can also be found in mast cells and eosinophils. It regulates the growth, differentiation, activation and survival of eosinophils. IL-5 contributes to eosinophil migration, tissue localization and function, and blocks their apoptosis. Eosinophils play a seminal role in the pathogenesis of allergic disease and asthma and in the defense against helminths and arthropods. The proliferation and differentiation of antigen-induced B lymphocytes and the production of IgA are also stimulated by IL-5. T_{H2} cytokines IL-4 and IL-5 play a central role in the induction of airway eosinophilia and AHR. It is a main player in inducing and sustaining the eosinophilic airway inflammation. IL-5 mediates its biological effects after binding to IL-5R, which is a membrane bound receptor. The receptor is composed of two chains, a ligand-specific α receptor (IL-5Rα) and a shared β receptor (IL-5Rβ). The β chain is also shared by IL-3 and GM-CSF, resulting in overlapping biological activity for these cytokines. The signaling through

IL-5R requires receptor-associated kinases. Two different signaling cascades associated with IL-5R include JAK/STAT and Ras/mitogens activated protein kinase (MAPK) pathways.

Interleukin-10

First identified as an inhibitor of IFN-γ synthesis in T_{H1} cells, IL-10 is an important immune regulatory cytokine. It is an anti-inflammatory cytokine that was first called human cytokine synthesis inhibitory factor. IL-10 is secreted by macrophages, T_{H2} cells and mast cells. Cytotoxic T-cells also release IL-10 to inhibit viral infection stimulated NK-cell activity. IL-10 is a 36-kDa dimer composed of two 160-aminoacid-residue-long chains. Its gene is located on chromosome 1 in humans and consists of five exons. IL-10 inhibits the synthesis of a number of cytokines involved in the inflammatory process including IL-2, IL-3, GM-CSF, TNF-α and IFN-γ.

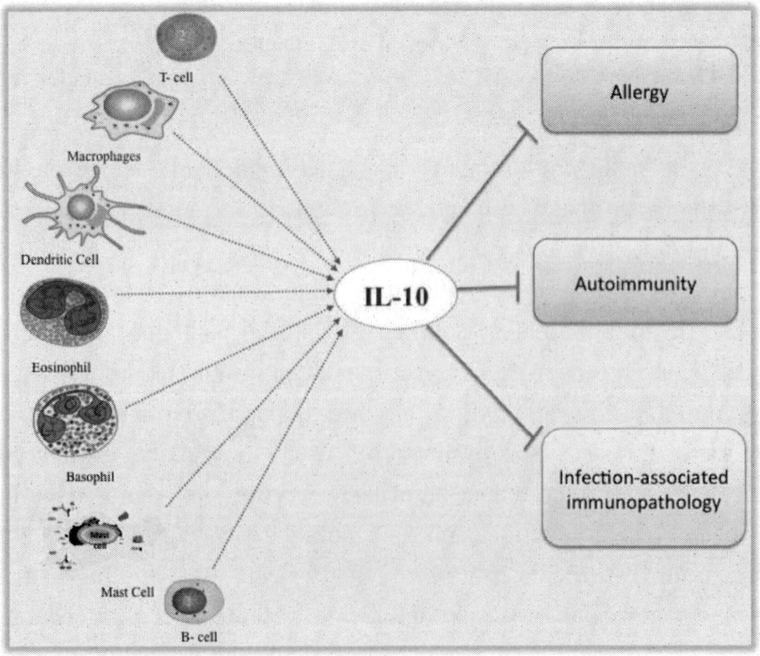

Figure 3.3. Role of interleukin 10 IL-10 in a number of immune responses.

Based on its cytokine-suppressing profile, it also functions as an inhibitor of T_{H1} cells and by virtue of inhibiting macrophages; it functions as an inhibitor of antigen presentation. Interestingly, IL-10 can promote the activity of mast cells, B-cells and certain T-cells (Figure 3.3).

Interleukin-11

IL-11, a member of the IL-6 super family, is produced by bone marrow stroma and activates B-cells, plasmacytomas, hepatocytes and megakaryocytes. The gene for IL-11 is located on chromosome 19. IL-11 induces acute-phase proteins, plays a role in bone cell proliferation and differentiation, increases platelet levels after chemotherapy and modulates antigen–antibody response. It promotes differentiation of progenitor B-cells and megakaryocytes. The recovery of neutrophils is accelerated by IL-11 after myelosuppressive therapy. IL-11 also possesses potent anti-inflammatory effects due to its ability to inhibit nuclear translocation of NF-κB. Additional biological effects of this cytokine include epithelial cell growth, osteoclastogenesis and inhibition of adipogenesis. The effects of IL-11 are mainly mediated via the IL-11 receptor chain. IL-11 forms a high-affinity complex in association with its receptor and associated proteins and induces gp130-dependentsignaling.

Interleukin-13

IL-13 belongs to the same α-helix super family as IL-4, and their genes are located12 kb apart on chromosome 5q31. It was originally identified for its effects on B-cells and monocytes, which included isotype switching from IgG to IgE, inhibition of inflammatory cytokines and enhancement of MHC class II expression. Initially, IL-13 appeared similar to IL-4 until its unique effector functions were recognized. Nevertheless, IL-13 and IL-4 have a number of overlapping effects (Figure 3.4). IL-13 also plays an essential role in resistance to most GI nematodes. It regulates mucus production, inflammation, fibrosis and tissue remodelling. IL-13 is a therapeutic target for a number of disease states including asthma, idiopathic pulmonary fibrosis, ulcerative colitis, cancer and others. Its signaling is mediated viaIL-4 type 2 receptor. The receptor consists of IL-α and IL-13Rα1 and IL-

13Rα2chains. IL-13 induces physiological changes in organs infected with parasites that are essential for eliminating the invading pathogen. In the gut, it induces a number of changes that make the surrounding environment of the parasite less hospitable, such as increasing contractions and hyper secretion of glycoproteins from gut epithelial cells. This results in the detachment of the parasites from the wall of the gut and their subsequent removal. IL-13 response in some instances may not resolve infection and may even be deleterious. For example, IL-13 may induce the formation of granulomas after organs such as the gut wall, lungs, liver and central nervous system are infected with the eggs of *Schistosoma mansoni*, which may lead to organ damage and could even be life threatening.

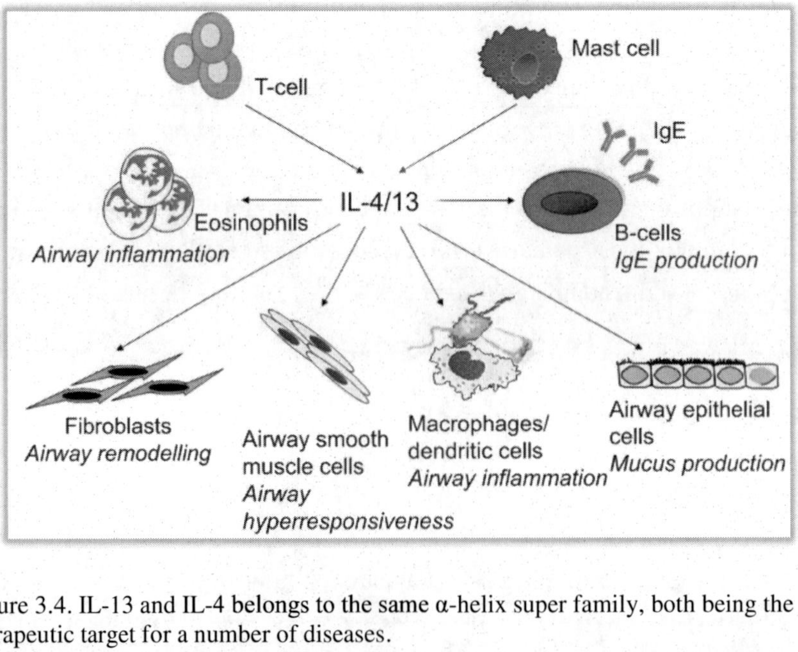

Figure 3.4. IL-13 and IL-4 belongs to the same α-helix super family, both being the therapeutic target for a number of diseases.

Interleukin-18

IL-18 is a member of the IL-1 family that promotes the production of various pro inflammatory mediators and plays a role in cancer and various infectious diseases (Figure 3.5). It was originally identified as IFN-γ-inducing factor and is produced by cells of both hematopoietic and non-hematopoietic lineages, including macrophages, dendritic cells, intestinal epithelial cells, synovial fibroblasts, keratinocytes, Kupffer cells, microglial cells and osteoblasts. The production of IL-18 is structurally homologous to that of IL-1β; it is produced as an inactive precursor of 24 kDa, which lacks a signal peptide. Endoprotease IL-1β-converting enzyme activates it after cleavingpro-IL-18, resulting in a biologically active cytokine. Caspase-1 plays an important role in the processing of IL-18, but is not exclusive since proteinase 3 can also perform the same function. IL-18 augments T- and NK-cell maturation, cytotoxicity and cytokine production. It stimulates T_H differentiation, promotes secretion of TNF-α, IFN-γ and GM-CSF and enhances NK-cell cytotoxicity by increasing FasL expression. IL-8-mediated neutrophil chemotaxis is promoted by IL-18 via its effects on TNF-α and IFN-γ, which are stimulatory in action. It plays an important role in maintaining synovial inflammation and inducing joint destruction in rheumatoid arthritis. In synovium of patients with rheumatoid arthritis, enhanced levels of TNF-α and IL-1are associated with augmented expression of IL-18. IL-18 also induces IL-4, IL-10 and IL-13 production, increases IgE expression on B-cells and in association with IL-2, it enhances.

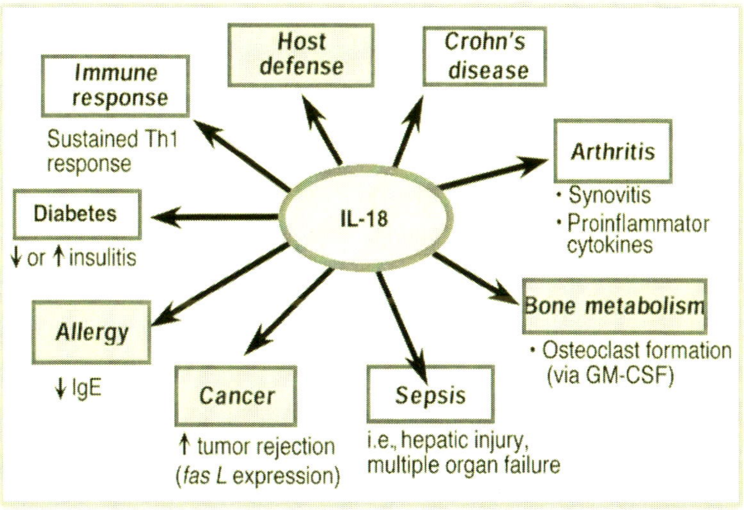

Figure 3.5. IL-18 promotes the production of various pro inflammatory mediators and plays a role in cancer and various infectious diseases.

Frequently Asked Questions

Q1. What do you understand by cascade induction of cytokines?

Answer: Cascade induction occurs when the action of one cytokine on a target cell induces that cell to produce one or more other cytokines, which in turn may induce other target cells to produce other cytokines.

Q2. Describe some properties of cytokines?

Answer: Cytokines bind to specific receptors on the membrane of target cells, triggering signal-transduction pathways that ultimately alter gene expression in the target cells. The susceptibility of the target cell to a particular cytokine is determined by the presence of specific membrane receptors. In general, the cytokines and their receptors exhibit very high affinity for each other, with dissociation constants ranging from 10^{-10} to 10^{-12} M. Because their affinities are so high, cytokines can mediate biological effects at picomolar concentrations

Q3. How does cytokines work?

Answer: While some important cytokine receptors lie outside the class I and class II families, the majority are included within these two families. As mentioned previously, class I and class II cytokine receptors lack signaling motifs (e.g., intrinsic tyrosine kinase domains). Yet, early observations demonstrated that one of the first events after the interaction of a cytokine with one of these receptors is a series of protein tyrosine phosphorylations. While these results were initially puzzling, they were explained when a unifying model emerged from studies of the molecular events triggered by binding of interferon gamma (IFN-γ) to its receptor, a member of the class II family.

Q4. What are the components of cytokine receptor?

Answer: The cytokine receptor is composed of separate subunits, an α chain required for cytokine binding and for signal transduction and a β chain necessary for signaling but with only a minor role in binding.

Q5. Describe the properties of IL-1?

Answer: Interleukin-1was originally discovered as a factor that induced fever, caused damage to joints and regulated bone marrow cells and lymphocytes, it was given several different names by various investigators. Later, the presence of two distinct proteins, IL-1α and IL-1β, was confirmed, which belong to a family of cytokines, the IL-1 superfamily. Ten ligands of IL-1 have been identified, termed IL-1F1 toIL-1F10. With the exception of IL-1F4, all of their genes map to the region of chromosome 2. IL-1 plays an important role in both innate and adaptive immunity and is a crucial mediator of the host inflammatory response in natural immunity. The major cell source of IL-1 is the activated mononuclear phagocyte. Other sources include dendritic cells, epithelial cells, endothelial cells, B cells, astrocytes, fibroblasts and large granular lymphocytes (LGL).

Q6. Discuss the functions of IL-1?

Answer: It produces the acute-phase response in response to infection. IL-1 induces fever as a result of bacterial and viral infections. It suppresses the appetite and induces muscle proteolysis, which may cause severe muscle "wasting" in patients with chronic infection. IL-1β causes the destruction of β cells leading to type 1 diabetes mellitus. It inhibits the function and promotes the apoptosis of pancreatic β cells. Activation of T-helper cells, resulting in IL-2 secretion, and B-cell activation are mediated by IL-1. It is a stimulator of fibroblast proliferation, which causes wound healing. Autoimmune diseases exhibit increased IL-1 concentrations.

Q7. Describe the properties of IL-2?

Answer: IL-2, a single polypeptide chain of 133 amino acid residues, is produced by immune regulatory cells that are principally T cells. When a helper T cell binds to an APC using CD28 and B7, CD4+ cells produce IL-2. IL-2 supports the proliferation and differentiation of any cell that has high-affinity IL-2 receptors. It is necessary for the activation of T cells. Resting T lymphocytes (un-stimulated) belonging to either the CD4+ or the CD8+ subsets possess few high-affinity IL-2 receptors, but following stimulation with specific antigen, there is a substantial increase in their numbers. The binding of IL-2 with its receptors on T cells induces their proliferation and differentiation.

MULTIPLE CHOICE QUESTIONS

Q1. Which among the following statements is correct for cytokines?

A. They are carbohydrates
B. They are glycoproteins
C. They are lipids
D. They are nucleic acids

Q2. The activity of cytokines was first observed in

A. 1950
B. 1940
C. Mid 1960
D. 1970

Q3. IL-13 belongs to the same α-helix superfamily as IL-4, and their genes are located12 kb apart on chromosome

A. 5q31
B. 6q31
C. 5p31
D. 6q31

Q4. IL-5 is secreted predominantly by

A. B cells
B. DC cells
C. Th2 cells
D. Th1 cells

Q5. Which among the following function of IL-5 on eosinophils is not correct?

A. Eosinophil migration
B. Tissue localization and function
C. Blocks their apoptosis of eosinophils.
D. Induces apoptosis of eosinophils

Q6. Which among the following statements is not correct for IL-13?

A. IL-13 and IL-4 have a number of overlapping effects.
B. IL-13 also playsan essential role in resistance to most GI nematodes.
C. It regulates mucus production, inflammation, fibrosis and tissue remodeling.
D. Its signaling is mediated viaIL-4 type 1 receptor.

Q7. Which among the following statements is Incorrect about IL-11?

A. IL-11, a member of the IL-6 superfamily
B. Produced by Thymus
C. Activates B cells
D. Induces acute-phase proteins
E. Plays a role in bone cell proliferation and differentiation

Q8. Which among the following statements is not correct for IL-2?

A. Produced by regulatory T cells
B. Necessary for the activation of T cells
C. Induces T cell proliferation and differentiation.
D. Produced by macrophages

Q9. Which among the following is the major growth factor for T lymphocytes?

A. IL-6
B. IL-2
C. IL-1
D. IL-10

Q10. The functions of IL-5 overlap with which of the following cytokine?

A. IL-6
B. IL-3
C. IL-8
D. IL-10

Q11. IL-4 has a number of overlapping effects with

A. IL-10
B. IL-13
C. IL-4
D. IL-2

Q12. Which among the following statements is NOT CORRECT for IL-10?

A. First identified as an inhibitor of IFN-γ synthesis in TH1 cells
B. IL-10 is an important immune-regulatory cytokine.
C. It is an anti-inflammatory cytokine
D. It is a pro-inflammatory cytokine

Q13. Which among the following is an anti-inflammatory cytokine?

A. IL-10
B. IL-12
C. IL-18
D. IL-1

Q14. Which among the following is not a pro-inflammatory cytokine?

A. IL-12
B. Interferon gamma
C. GM-csf
D. IL-10

Q15. Which among the following statements is not correct for IL-1?

A. It promotes the function and inhibits the apoptosis of pancreatic β cells.

B. Activates T-helper cells

C. B-cell activation

D. It is a stimulator of fibroblast proliferation

Answer Key

1(B), 2(C), 3(A), 4(C), 5(D), 6(D), 7(B), 8(D), 9(B), 10(B), 11(B), 12(D), 13(A), 14(D), 15(A).

ASSIGNMENTS

Q1. Describe the properties of cytokines in detail?

Q2. Explain the effects of IL-2 on the immune cells?

Q3. Explain the effects of IL-10 on the immune cells?

Q4. Describe the properties of IL-13?

Q5. What do you understand by pleiotropy of cytokines?

REFERENCES

Arend WP, Dayer JM. 1990. Cytokines and cytokine inhibitors or antagonists in rheumatoidarthritis. *Arthritis Rheumat.* 33:305–315.

Asadullah K, Sterry W, Volk HD. 2003. Interleukin-10 therapy – Review of a new approach. *Pharmacol Rev.* 55:241–269.

Atkins MB. 2002. Interleukin-2: Clinical applications. *Semin Oncol.* 29:12–17.

Auron PE, Webb AC, Rosenwassser LJ, Mucci SF, et al. 1984. Nucleotide sequence of humanmonocyte interleukin 1 precursor CDA. *Proc Nat Acad Sci USA*. 81:7907–7911.

Balkwill FR, Burke F. The cytokine network. *Immunol Today.* 1989;10:299–304.

Becknell B, Caligiuri MA. 2005. Interleukin 2 and interleukin 15, and their roles in human naturalkiller cells. *Adv Immunol.* 86:209–239.

Bhatia M, Davenport V, Cairo MS. 2007. The role of interleukin-11 to prevent chemotherapyinducedcytopenia in patients with solid tumors, lymphomas, acute myeloid leukemia andbone marrow failure syndromes. *Leuk Lymph*. 48:9–15.

Bhokta NR, Woodruff PG. Human asthma phenotypes: from the clinic, to cytokines, and back again. *Immunol Rev*. 2011;242:220–32.

Bienvenu J, Monneret G, Fabien N, Revillard JP. The clinical usefulness of the measurement of cytokines. *Clinical Chemistry and Laboratory Medicine.* 2000;38:267–85.

Bouchner BS, Klunk DA, Sterbinsky SA, Coffman RL, et al. 1995. IL-13 selectively inducesvascular cell adhesion molecule-1 expression in human endothelial cells. *J Immuno*. 154:799–803.

Bradding P, Roberts JA, Britten KM, Montefort S, et al. 1994. Interleukin-4, -5, and -6 and tumornecrosis factor-alpha in normal and asthmatic airways: Evidence for the human mast cell as asource of these cytokines. *Am J Respir Cell Mol Biol.* 10:471–480.

Brunet M. Cytokines as predictive biomarkers of alloreactivity. *Clin Chim Acta*. 2012;413:1354–8.

Buetler B, Greenwald D, Hulmes JD, Chang M, et al. 1985. Identity of tumor necrosis factor andthe macrophage-secreted factor cachectin. *Nature.* 316:552–554.

Burska A, Boissinot M, Ponchel F. Cytokines as biomarkers in rheumatoid arthritis. *Mediators Inflamm*. 2014;2014:545493.

Candace A. Gilbert, et al. Cytokines, Obesity, and Cancer: New Insights on Mechanisms Linking Obesity to Cancer Risk and Progression. *Annu. Rev. Med*. 2013. 64:45–57.

Catalfamo M, Le SC, Lane HC. The role of cytokines in the pathogenesis and treatment of HIV infection. *Cytokine Growth Factor Rev.* 2012;23:207–14.

Charo IF, Romsohoff RM. 2006. The many roles of chemokines and chemokines receptors ininflammation. *NEJM.* 354:610–621.

Chaouat G, Dubanchet S, Ledée N. Cytokines: Important for implantation?. *J Assist Reprod Genet.* 2007;24(11):491–505. doi:10.1007/s10815-007-9142-9.

Chikkaveeraiah BV, Bhirde AA, Morgan NY, Eden HS, Chen X. Electrochemical Immunosensors for Detection of Cancer Protein Biomarkers. *ACS Nano.* 2012;6:6546–61.

Chen HF, Shew JY, Ho HN, Hsu WL, Yang YS (October 1999). "Expression of leukemia inhibitory factor and its receptor in preimplantation embryos." *Fertil. Steril.* 72 (4): 713–9.

Dimitrov, Dimiter S. (2012). "Therapeutic Proteins." *Methods in Molecular Biology.* 899. pp. 1–26.

Dinarello CA (August 2000). "Proinflammatory cytokines." *Chest.* 118 (2): 503–8.

Dowlati Y, Herrmann N, Swardfager W, Liu H, Sham L, Reim EK, Lanctôt KL (March 2010). "A meta-analysis of cytokines in major depression." *Biol. Psychiatry.* 67 (5): 446–57.

Giovanni Germano, et al. Cytokines as a key component of cancer-related inflammation. *Cytokine* 43 (2008) 374–379.

Gui T, Shimokado A, Sun Y, Akasaka T, Muragaki Y. Diverse roles of macrophages in atherosclerosis: from inflammatory biology to biomarker discovery. *Mediators Inflammation.* 2012;693083:14.

Gullestad L, Ueland T, Vinge LE, Finsen A, Yndestad A, Aukrust P. Inflammatory Cytokines in Heart Failure: Mediators and Markers. *Cardiology.* 2012;122:23–35.

Horst Ibelgaufts. Recombinant cytokines in *Cytokines & Cells Online Pathfinder Encyclopedia* Version 31.4 (Spring/Summer 2013 Edition).

Iarlori C, Gambi D, Reale M. *Parkinson's disease and cytokines.* Science Publishers, Inc; 2011. pp. 343–55.

Khan MM. Role of cytokines. In *Immunopharmacology* 2016 (pp. 57-92). Springer, Cham.

Key LL, Rodriguiz RM, Willi SM, Wright NM, Hatcher HC, Eyre DR, Cure JK, Griffin PP, Ries WL (June 1995). "Long-term treatment of osteopetrosis with recombinant human interferon gamma." *N. Engl. J. Med.* 332 (24): 1594–9.

Lee DW, Faubel S, Edelstein CL. Cytokines in acute kidney injury (AKI) *Clin Nephrol.* 2011;76:165–73.

Levine JE, Paczesny S, Sarantopoulos S. Clinical Applications for Biomarkers of Acute and Chronic Graft-versus-Host Disease. *Biol Blood Marrow Transplant.* 2012;18:S116–S24.

Locksley RM, Killeen N, Lenardo MJ (February 2001). "The TNF and TNF receptor superfamilies: integrating mammalian biology." *Cell.* 104 (4): 487–501.

Long TM, Raufman JP. The diagnostic and prognostic role of cytokines in colon cancer. *Gastrointest Cancer: Targets Ther*. 2011;1:27–39.

Lotrich F. Inflammatory cytokines, growth factors, and depression. *Curr Pharm Des.* 2012;18:5920–35.

Makhija R, Kingsnorth AN (2002). "Cytokine storm in acute pancreatitis." *J Hepatobiliary Pancreat Surg.* 9 (4): 401–10.

Mukai K, Tsai M, Saito H, Galli SJ. Mast cells as sources of cytokines, chemokines, and growth factors. *Immunol Rev*. 2018;282(1):121–150.

Prieto GA, Cotman CW. Cytokines and cytokine networks target neurons to modulate long-term potentiation. *Cytokine Growth Factor Rev.* 2017;34:27–33.

Reinhart K, Bauer M, Riedemann NC, Hartog CS. New approaches to sepsis: molecular diagnostics and biomarkers. *Clin Microbiol Rev.* 2012;25:609–34.

Rose NR. Critical Cytokine Pathways to Cardiac Inflammation. *J Interferon Cytokine Res.* 2011;31:705–10.

Rusling JF, Kumar CV, Gutkind JS, Patel V. Measurement of biomarker proteins for point-of-care early detection and monitoring of cancer. *Analyst* (Cambridge, U K) 2010;135:2496–511.

Saito S (2001). "Cytokine cross-talk between mother and the embryo/placenta." *J. Reprod. Immunol.* 52 (1–2): 15–33.

Schenk T, Irth H, Marko-Varga G, Edholm LE, Tjaden UR, van dGJ. Potential of on-line micro-LC immunochemical detection in the bioanalysis of cytokines. *J Pharm Biomed Anal.* 2001; 26: 975–85.

Schmitz ML, Weber A, Roxlau T, Gaestel M, Kracht M. Signal integration, crosstalk mechanisms and networks in the function of inflammatory cytokines. *Biochim Biophys Acta, Mol Cell Res.* 2011; 1813: 2165–75.

Schett G, Elewaut D, McInnes IB, Dayer J-M, Neurath MF. How cytokine networks fuel inflammation: Toward a cytokine-based disease taxonomy. *Nat Med.* 2013; 19: 822–4.

Striz I, Brabcova E, Kolesar L, Sekerkova A. Cytokine networking of innate immunity cells: a potential target of therapy. *Clin Sci.* 2014; 126:593–612.

Swardfager W, Lanctôt K, Rothenburg L, Wong A, Cappell J, Herrmann N (November 2010). "A meta-analysis of cytokines in Alzheimer's disease." *Biol. Psychiatry.* 68 (10): 930–41.

Velluto L, Iarlori C, Gambi D, Reale M. *Cytokines and Alzheimer's disease.* Science Publishers, Inc; 2011. pp. 329–42.

Vlahopoulos SA, Cen O, Hengen N, Agan J, Moschovi M, Critselis E, Adamaki M, Bacopoulou F, Copland JA, Boldogh I, Karin M, Chrousos GP (August 2015). "Dynamic aberrant NF-κB spurs tumorigenesis: a new model encompassing the microenvironment." *Cytokine Growth Factor Rev.* 26 (4): 389–403.

Wakita T, Shintani F, Yagi G, Asai M, Nozawa S. Combination of inflammatory cytokines increases nitrite and nitrate levels in the paraventricular nucleus of conscious rats. *Brain Res.* 2001; 905: 12–20.

Woodman RC, Erickson RW, Rae J, Jaffe HS, Curnutte JT (March 1992). "Prolonged recombinant interferon-gamma therapy in chronic granulomatous disease: evidence against enhanced neutrophil oxidase activity." *Blood.* 79 (6): 1558–62.

Zhu H, Wang Z, Yu J, et al. (March 2019). "Role and mechanisms of cytokines in the secondary brain injury after intracerebral hemorrhage." *Prog Neurobiol.* 178:101610.

In: Cytokines and Their Therapeutic Potential ISBN: 978-1-53617-017-7
Editor: Manzoor Ahmad Mir

Chapter 4

THERAPEUTIC CYTOKINES

Nissar A. Wani, Umar Mehraj, Safura Nisar, Bashir Ahmad Sheikh, Syed Suhail Hamdani, Hina Qayoom and Manzoor Ahmad Mir*

Department of Bioresources, School of Biological Sciences, University of Kashmir, Srinagar Jammu and Kashmir, India

ABSTRACT

Cytokines help regulate and direct the immune system. Cells release cytokines, which act as messengers to other cells, telling them when and where to launch an immune response. These are low molecular mass (generally less than 30 KDa) soluble proteins/glycoproteins, non-immunoglobulin in nature and do not include the peptides and steroid hormones of the endocrine system. These proteins assist in regulating the development of immune effector cells and some cytokines possess direct effector functions of their own. Cytokines bind to specific receptors on the membrane of target cells, triggering signal-transduction pathways that ultimately alter gene expression in the target cells. The susceptibility of the target cell to a particular cytokine is determined by the presence of specific membrane receptors. In general, the cytokines and their receptors exhibit

* Corresponding Author's Email: drmanzoor@kashmiruniversity.ac.in.

very high affinity for each other with the dissociation constants ranging from 10^{-10} to 10^{-12} M. Because of their high affinities, cytokines can mediate biological effects even at Pico molar concentrations. A particular cytokine may bind to receptors on the membrane of the same cell that secreted it, exerting autocrine action or it may bind to receptors on a target cell in close proximity to the producer cell exerting paracrine action or in a few cases, it may bind to target cells in distant body parts exerting endocrine action.

Keywords: infection, HIV, immunodeficiency, clinical therapies, cytokines, factors, administration, conjugates, recombinant, transplants, diseases, immunotherapy, melanoma, hematopoiesis, cancer, kidney, tuberculosis, receptors

OBJECTIVES

- To get a basic understanding about therapeutic cytokines.
- Describe working of cytokines and the effects they induce.
- Understanding the role of cytokines in immunoregulation.
- Discuss the use and advantage of using cytokines in therapy.
- Advanced research studies being conducted in of therapeutic cytokines.

INTRODUCTION

As the researches advance and tools are improving to understand the immune system, more is being learned about cytokines. There is an increased interest in harnessing the language of the immune system to direct its responses and improve health. This research holds a great potential, in realizing that it will likely be riddled with failed experiments and confounding results. Cytokine therapy is not merely a tool of the future, but years from the grasp of our medicine cabinets. To the contrary, several cytokine therapies are now routinely used by many people living with HIV.

IL-2 in combination with anti-HIV therapy are expected within the next 2-3 years. Hopefully in the next few years we may have therapies for various diseases by using cytokines alone or in combination. Cytokines are general immune system boosters. They rally our immune system's defences to fight damaged cells. Targeted immune-therapies on the other hand act on specific proteins on particular cells. They change the way that immune cells interact with damaged cells and thus make it possible for our existing immune system to fight the various diseases without giving any boosts. The availability of purified cloned cytokines and soluble cytokine receptors provides the prospect for specific clinical therapies to modulate the immune response. A few cytokines—notably, interferons and colony stimulating factors, such as GM-CSF, have proven to be therapeutically useful. However, despite the promise of cytokines as powerful mediators of immune and other biological responses, not many have made their way into clinical practice. A number of factors are likely to raise difficulties in adapting cytokines for safe and effective routine medical use. One of these is the need to maintain effective dose levels over a clinically significant period of time.

During an immune response, interacting cells produce sufficiently high concentrations of cytokines in the vicinity of target cells, but achieving such local concentrations when cytokines must be administered systemically for clinical treatment is difficult. In addition, cytokines often have a very short half-life, so that continuous administration may be required. For example, recombinant human IL-2 has a half-life of only 7–10 min when administered intravenously. Finally, cytokines are extremely potent biological response modifiers and they can cause unpredictable and undesirable side effects.

The side effects from administration of recombinant IL-2, for instance, range from mild e.g., fever, chills, diarrhea, and weight gain to serious condition like: anemia, thrombocytopenia, shock, respiratory distress, and coma. Despite these difficulties, the promise of cytokines for clinical medicine is great and efforts to develop safe and effective cytokine-related strategies continue, particularly in areas such as inflammation, cancer therapy, and modification of the immune response during organ transplantation, infectious disease, and allergy. Some specific examples of various approaches being explored include cytokine receptor blockade and the use of cytokine analogs and cytokine-toxin conjugates. For instance, proliferation of activated T_H cells and activation of T_C cells can be blocked by anti-TAC, a monoclonal antibody that binds to a subunit of the high-affinity. IL-2 receptor. Administration of anti-TAC has prolonged the survival of heart transplants in rats. Similar results have been obtained with IL-2 analogs that retain their ability to bind the IL-2 receptor but have lost their biological activity. Such analogs have been produced by site-directed mutagenesis of cloned IL-2 genes. In the end, cytokines conjugated to various toxins e.g., the chain of diphtheria toxin have been shown to diminish rejection of kidney and heart transplants in animals. Such conjugates containing IL-2 selectively bind to and kill activated T_H cells. A particular cytokine may bind to receptors on the membrane of the same cell that secreted it, exerting autocrine action or it may bind to receptors on a target cell in close proximity to the producer cell exerting paracrine action or in a few cases, it may bind to target cells in distant body parts exerting endocrine action.

Cytokines regulate the intensity and duration of the immune response by stimulating or inhibiting the activation, proliferation and/or differentiation of various cells and by regulating the secretion of antibodies or other cytokines. Cytokines exhibit the attributes of pleiotropy, redundancy, synergy, antagonism and cascade induction which permit them to regulate cellular activity in a coordinated, interactive way. A cytokine that has different biological effects on different target cells has a pleiotropic action. Two or more cytokines that mediate similar functions are said to be redundant. Cytokine synergism occurs when the combined effect of two cytokines on cellular activity is greater than the additive effects of the individual cytokines. In some cases cytokines exhibit antagonism which is the effects of one cytokine inhibits or offset the effects of another cytokine. Cytokines share many properties with hormones and growth factors; the distinction between them is often blurred. All of these are secreted soluble factors that elicit their biological effects at picomolar concentrations by binding to receptors on target cells. Growth factors tend to be produced constitutively while cytokines and hormones are secreted in response to discrete stimuli but unlike hormones which act long range, cytokines act over a short distance mostly.

Clinical Functions of Cytokines

Although a variety of cells can secrete cytokines, the two principal producers are the T_H cell and the macrophage. Cytokines released from these two cell types activate an entire network of interacting cells. Among the numerous physiologic responses that require cytokine involvement are development of cellular and humoral immune responses, induction of the inflammatory response, regulation of haematopoiesis, control of cellular proliferation and differentiation and the healing of wounds. Besides regulating immune responses cytokine target various types of tissues and cells in the body and regulate a number of processes like Chemotaxis, apoptosis, necrosis, proliferation, differentiation and metabolic activation (Figure 4).

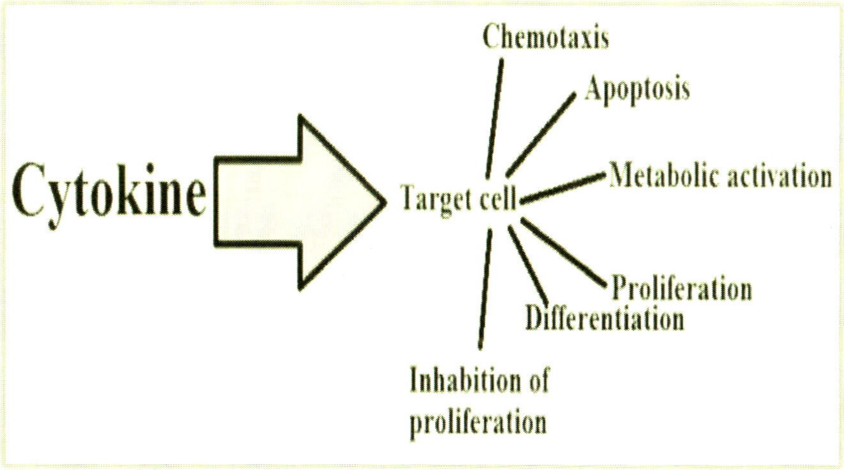

Figure 4.1. Cytokine target various types of tissues and cells in the body and regulate a number of processes.

Role of Cytokines in Immune Responses

Cytokines are involved in a staggeringly broad array of biological activities including innate immunity, adaptive immunity, inflammation and haematopoiesis. The main cytokines that have a role in the innate responses are: IL-1, IL-6, IL-12, IL-16, TNF α, INF α and β. The IL-1, IL-6 and IL-12 activate the monocytes-macrophages and NK cells. Tumour necrosis factor is the main trigger of the inflammatory response. T_H cells exert most of their helper functions through secreted cytokines. Although CTLs also secrete cytokines, their array of cytokines generally is more restricted than that of T_H cells. Antigen stimulation of T_H cells in the presence of certain cytokines can lead to the generation of subpopulations of helper T-cells known as T_H1 and T_H2. Each subset displays characteristic and different profiles of cytokine secretion. The main cytokines that have a role in adaptive immune response are: IL-2, IL-4, IL-5, TGF β and IFN γ.

Cytokines and Immunotherapy

Advances in the understanding of the role of cytokines in immune and inflammatory disorders have led to the development of cytokine-based therapies. Therapies have been developed with the express aim to block/inhibit or restore the activity of specific cytokines. Cytokines delivered by gene therapy and antisense oligonucleotide treatment are also being assessed. Currently, the most utilized approach to cytokine therapy is that of blocking or neutralizing cytokine action with monoclonal antibodies (mAbs). Drugs that block inflammatory cytokines, such as tumour necrosis factor TNF-α, are among the most successful therapeutics approved for clinical use.

Cytokine Immunotherapy

Immunotherapy is a medical term defined as the "treatment of disease by inducing, enhancing, or suppressing an immune response." The active agents of immunotherapy are collectively called immune modulators. They are a diverse array of recombinant, synthetic and natural preparations, often cytokines, such as granulocyte colony-stimulating factor (G-CSF), interferons, imiquimod and cellular membrane fractions from bacteria are already licensed for use in patients. Others including IL-2, IL-7, IL-12, various chemokines, synthetic cytosine phosphate-guanosine (CpG), oligodeoxynucleotides and glucans are currently being investigated extensively in clinical and preclinical studies. The field of cytokines is of age in the late 1970s with the introduction of molecular biological approaches that resulted first in the cloning of IFNs, initially IFN-β by Tada Taniguchi and IFN-α by both Charles Weissman's group and David Goeddel's colleagues.

By the mid-1980s, there was a plethora of well-defined cytokines and cytokine receptors that could be unambiguously studied, using molecular tools, such as cDNA probes, and antibodies that had been produced to recognize the pure recombinant proteins. All this was a long way from the 1960s and 1970s, when all researchers had were many uncharacterized bioactivities in cell supernatants termed simply by activity, e.g., lymphocyte-activating factor, macrophage-activating factor, and leukocyte pyrogen. All the tools available by the mid-1980s enabled researchers to assess the expression of cytokines in physiologic and pathologic states. The up regulated expression of cytokines in many different disease states led to an investigation of their role in the pathogenesis of disease (Fig 4.1), and the articles in this Review Series barely scratch the surface of the plethora of information available now.

As cytokines are potent rate-limiting extracellular molecules, they are excellent targets for the products of the biotechnology industry, namely monoclonal antibodies and antibody-like receptor: Fc fusion proteins. These form the most specific therapeutics, more specific than small molecule organic chemicals, due to the greater surface of interaction of receptors and antibodies with their targets.

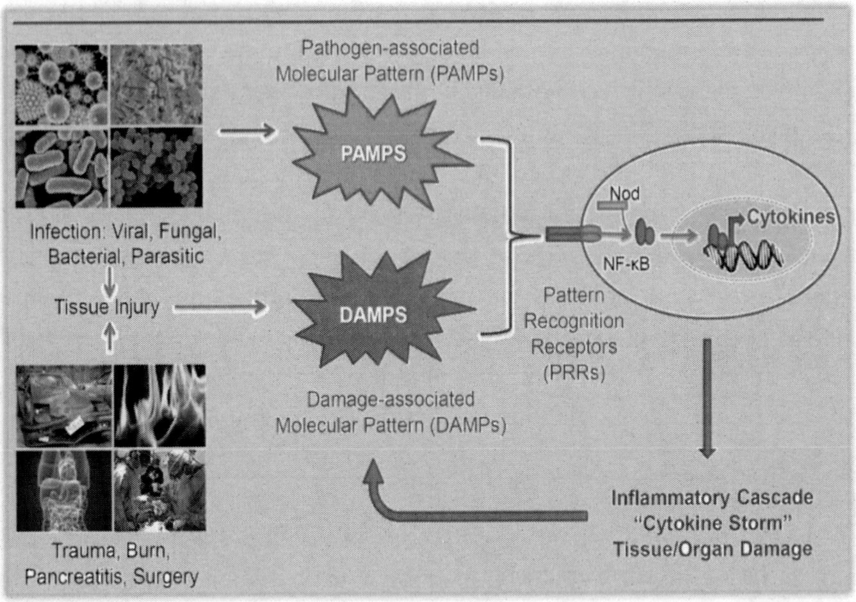

Figure 4.2. Excessive production of pro-inflammatory cytokines, contribute to the immune pathogenesis of a number of diseases.

Cytokines in Immune and Inflammatory Disorders

Cytokines mediate a wide variety of biological activities that are relevant to autoimmune diseases, including inflammation induced by an immune response, as well as tissue repair and remodelling. The roles of different cytokines in autoimmune diseases have been widely studied. It has become clear that excessive production of pro-inflammatory cytokines, as well as the relative paucity of regulatory cytokines contribute to the immune pathogenesis of these diseases. Restoring optimal cytokine balance may have therapeutic value that theoretically could be achieved either by blocking inflammatory cytokines or inducing or providing anti-inflammatory ones. Rheumatoid arthritis is a common autoimmune disease and the first big success of anti-cytokine therapy, in the form of TNF-α blockade, was demonstrated in this disease, and it has now been repeatedly shown that blocking this single cytokine has marked beneficial effects on all aspects of disease activity and can prevent further joint destruction. In addition, it has been determined that several other important chronic diseases respond to TNF-α blockade. Due to the ease of performing clinical trials with well-established protocols, multiple cytokine blockade clinical trials have been performed in severe RA. These clinical trials have had variable success, and it is not understood why in this disease, as in many others, there are differences between results in animal models, where many anti-cytokine therapies are very effective, and the human disease, treatment of which is proving more challenging. For example, in the mouse model of RA, blockade of IL-1 is just as beneficial as TNF-α blockade, sometimes more so but while IL-1 blockade in the form of IL-1 receptor antagonist (IL-1Ra) is effective and approved in RA, it is a less potent therapeutic approach than TNF-α blockade and hence has not been as extensively used in the clinic. Not known, the effect of blockade of many other cytokines that might have an important role in the pathogenesis of RA, including IL-12/23, IL-17, IL-18, IL-27, and IL-32.

Multiple sclerosis (MS) is an important neurodegenerative disease in which inflammation and cytokines are prominent in the affected tissue. In multiple sclerosis (MS) activated auto-reactive T-cells, B-cells, and other mononuclear cells cross the blood–brain barrier and enter the central nervous system (CNS). These mononuclear cell infiltrates, together with resident CNS cells, can cause injury to oligodendrocytes and myelin. There are at least four clinical subtypes of this disease. The relapsing-remitting form is the most common (80–85%) and is characterized by acute attacks (relapses) followed by remissions. Human beta interferon (IFN-β) has been demonstrated to modulate many of these processes. Two forms of IFN-β are in clinical use: IFN-β1a and IFN-β1b. Despite some differences in their pharmacologic properties they have similar clinical effects. Seven large, randomized placebo-controlled trials have demonstrated clinical efficacy in both relapsing-remitting (three studies) MS and secondary progressive (four studies) MS. These trials have consistently demonstrated that both forms of

IFN-β reduce disease activity by reducing clinical attack rate and magnetic resonance imaging (MRI) activity measures. IFN-β treatment seems also to improve disease severity in MS; however these data are less convincing. The more recent clinical studies have focused on the impact of dose and optimal dosing frequency. The currently available data suggest that higher dose and/or more frequent administration may increase the efficacy of IFN-β treatment in MS.

Cytokine Therapy for Treating Malignancies

Cytokine therapy has proven to be a novel therapeutic approach in treating patients with advanced malignancies. The purpose of this type of therapy is to manipulate the immune response in such a way as to generate the appropriate immune effector cells to eradicate solid tumours. Cytokine therapy is administrated only after the conventional form of therapies have been performed such as chemotherapy, radiotherapy, and surgery. Various regimens of cytokine administration have been implemented in eradicating solid tumours in patients with melanoma and renal cell cancer. There have been clinical trials executed involving the administration of interferon-gamma INF-γ, interferon-alpha INF-α, Interleukin-2, tumour necrosis factor-alpha TNF-α, and Interleukin-12. Advances in cytokine therapy have been thwarted by the relatively high level of toxicity associated with the administration of cytokines. Common toxicities include nausea, vomiting, fever/chills, fatigue, and headache. Dose escalation of a particular cytokine halts once three patients at particular dose level experience grade three toxicity. The maximum tolerated dose of the cytokine is designated as the preceding dose. In turn, determining the schedule of treatment is another challenge at hand for clinicians. Partial or complete tumour regression has been noted in some clinical trials which offer hope in finding the appropriate cytokine or combination of cytokines and dose level to effectively treat advanced malignancies without being too toxic to the patient (Figure 4.2).

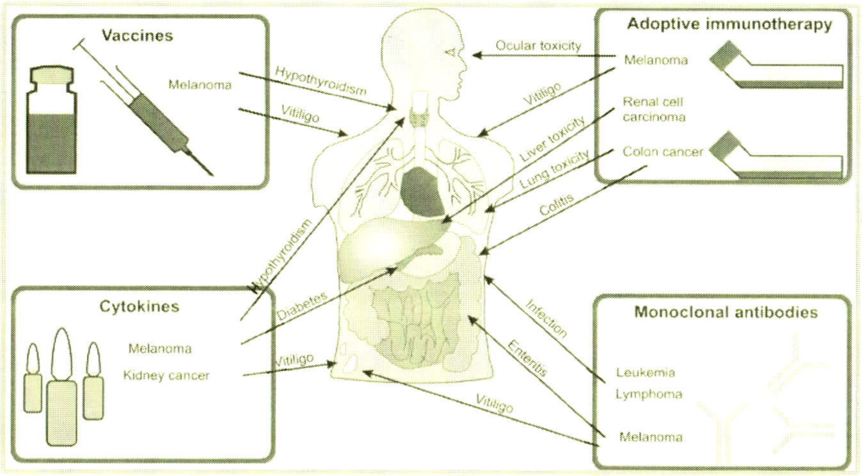

Figure 4.3. An appropriate cytokine or combination of cytokines that can effectively treat advanced malignancies without being too toxic to the patient.

Cytokines to Treat Skin Cancer

Cytokines can be used as a primary treatment or adjuvant treatment for skin cancer. They can be used alone or as part of a combination treatment approach called bio chemotherapy. Primary treatment is the first treatment given for cancer. It is usually chosen based upon the stage and type of cancer, other genetic factors for the individual patient, and is considered in relation to other treatment options available. Adjuvant therapy is an additional cancer treatment that is given after the primary treatment. Adjuvant therapy can help lower the risk that the cancer comes back. Bio chemotherapy is the combination of interleukin-2, interferon, and chemotherapy. IL-2 is a cytokine that activates our immune system. Our body makes IL-2 naturally in small amounts. Taking larger amounts of IL-2 as medication, it gives our immune system a boost. IL-2 tells our body to make more T-cells and Natural Killer cells. T-cells (T-lymphocytes) and Natural Killer cells are white blood cells. They fight cancer and infection. IL-2 makes T-cells better at killing cancer cells. IL-2 also increases production of interferon, another immune system booster. Interferon-alpha INF-α, is a cytokine that also activates our immune system. Our body makes interferon naturally in small amounts. Taking larger amounts of interferon-alpha, INF-α as medication can give our immune system a boost. Interferon is a signalling molecule; it does not attack cancer cells directly, instead, it attaches to a receptor on the surface of a cell and sets off a chain of events inside the cell. Peg interferon alpha-2b is a cytokine that is made in a lab and taken as a medication. Peg interferon alpha-2b is also called by the brand name Sylatron. It is made by combining man-made interferon-alpha INF-α, with a chemical called polyethylene glycol (PEG). Adding PEG keeps the interferon-alpha INF-α longer in our body. The result is that peg interferon can be given less frequently than interferon-alpha-3a.

Cytokine Therapy for High-Risk Stage II Melanoma

In stage II melanoma, the cancer is not spread beyond the skin tumour. However, thick skin tumours are considered at high-risk for recurrence. Interferon-alpha INF-α, a cytokine may be used as adjuvant as treatment for thick stage II melanoma.

Cytokine Therapy for Stage III Melanoma

In stage III melanoma, the cancer spreads to the lymph nodes. Options for adjuvant treatment for stage III cancer include interferon-alpha INF-α, peg interferon, or bio-chemotherapy. Satellite or in-transit tumours are found near the main tumour. They may be treated by injecting interleukin-2 or interferon directly into them.

Cytokine Therapy for Stage IV (Metastatic) Melanoma

Metastatic melanoma is when the cancer is spread over to distant parts of the body. High-dose interleukin-2 or bio-chemotherapy can be used to treat metastatic melanoma. It is usually used if other treatments are not working.

Cytokine Therapy for Kaposi Sarcoma

Interferon-alpha INF-α, is used to treat some patients with Kaposi sarcoma. It works best for patients with no systemic symptoms, limited lymph node disease, and fairly good immune function.

Role of Cytokines in HIV Treatment

HIV infection targets the immune system leading to a state of immunodeficiency in setting of immune activation. The molecular mechanisms causing the pathogenesis of HIV infection are still incompletely understood and are probably a composite of multiple factors. The acute phase of HIV infection or SIV infected rhesus macaques (RM) is characterized by a substantial drop in peripheral CD4 T-cell counts and a substantial depletion of memory CD4+ CCR5+ T-cells. In the chronic phase, a continued decline of CD4 T-cells associated with ongoing HIV replication leads to the development of AIDS. Several methods have been tried to stimulate inactive cells infected with HIV. Some studies have shown that the immune system chemical messenger interleukin-7 (IL-7) and a protein kinase activator called prostratin can trigger resting CD4 T-cells to produce HIV without stimulating activation of all T-cells.

Interleukin-7 appears to work at earlier stages, stimulating production of T-cells in the bone marrow and encouraging their maturation in the thymus, than the more thoroughly investigated IL-2, which mainly increases T-cell numbers by promoting proliferation of mature T-cells. The cytokine that has received the most attention as an immune restoration therapy for people with HIV is a recombinant version of interleukin-2 (IL-2). Naturally produced by the body, IL-2 encourages the proliferation of CD4 T-cells. Manufactured versions of IL-2, given by injection, trigger the production of CD4 cells by mimicking the body's own inflammatory response. IL-2 can thus produce significant boosts in CD4 cell count levels, as demonstrated in many clinical trials, but it has yet to find a well-defined clinical use outside the experimental setting.

Therapy with Interferons

Interferons are an extraordinary group of proteins whose antiviral activity led to their discovery almost 50 years ago. The discovery of interferons was a result of research by Isaacs & Lindeman in the field of viral interference, the ability of an active or inactivated virus to interfere with the growth of an unrelated virus. Until 1957, viral interference had been considered to be due directly to the action of one virus on the pathologic activity of a second agent. The Mill Hill group demonstrated that most instances of viral interference were a result of the induction by the interfering agent of cellular products, interferons, later shown to be proteins that in turn activate a number of genes responsible for the biologic effects ascribed to the interferons in addition to their antiviral activity. Interest in the possible clinical application of interferons picked up in the mid-1970s when sufficient quantities of human IFN-α became available for small studies, in great part to the efforts of Cantell and his co-workers, who were responsible for blood banking in Finland, and had previously carried out research on interferons.

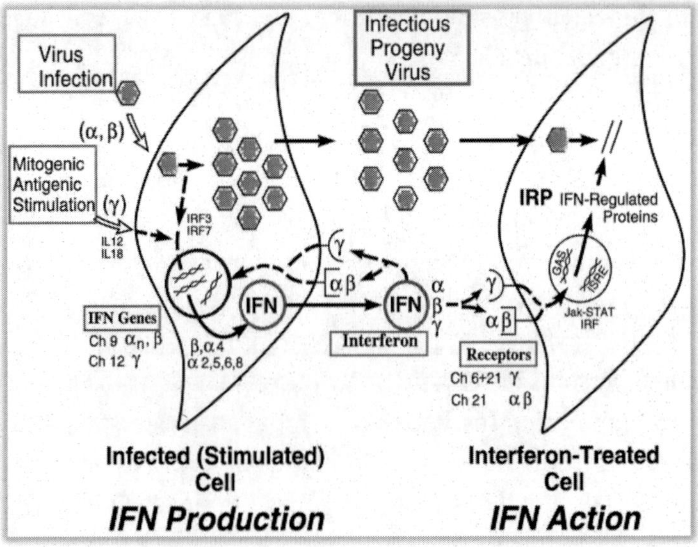

Figure 4.4. Interferons to treat chronic virus infections in patients.

Purified, but not pure preparations of human IFN-α, obtained from the white blood cells, buffy coat of donated blood, were supplied by Cantell's group for a number of clinical experiments, many of which had promising results in studies on the prevention of common colds and the treatment of several herpes virus infections, such as herpes kerato conjunctivitis and varicella-zoster infections, shingles and chicken-pox. When treatment with interferon in tissue culture was found to inhibit chronic infections with mouse leukaemia viruses, it seemed reasonable to try to treat chronic virus infections in patients with interferons, and indeed clinical studies employing IFN-α in chronic hepatitis B virus (HBV) infections yielding very promising results (Fig: 4.3). In 1982 Jacobs et al. treated 10 multiple sclerosis (MS) patients with partially purified human IFN-β, administered by lumbar puncture, and reported a significant decrease in the frequency of the periodic exacerbations characteristic of MS.

Cytokines as Immune-Modulators in Tuberculosis Therapy

The use of cytokines for therapeutic purposes is limited by their high cost and toxicity. Nevertheless, the emergence of extensively drug-resistant tuberculosis (XDR TB), for which chemotherapy is ineffective, has again made cytokine-based therapy attractive as one of the last available options. The results of clinical trials treating pulmonary tuberculosis with cytokines have not been encouraging, making it clear that therapeutic strategies utilizing a single cytokine are inadequate. To develop effective cytokine-based XDR TB therapies, more basic research will be needed to achieve a better understanding of how cytokines promote a successful immune response. There are already several patents involving cytokines for therapeutic use, in the hope of stimulating the immune system in a variety of infectious diseases, including tuberculosis. The validity of these patents needs to be reassessed from a clinical standpoint, and new applications of patents concerning cytokines potentially useful in XDR TB treatment should be encouraged.

Table 4.1. Cytokine based therapies in clinical use

Agent	Nature of agent	Clinical application
Enbrel	Chimeric TNF-receptor/IgG constant region	Rheumatoid arithritis
Remicade	Monoclonal antibody against TNF-α receptor	Rheumatoid arithritis
Interferon α-2a	Antiviral cytokine	Hepatitis B Hairy cell leukemia Kaposi's sarcoma
Interferon α-2b	Antiviral cytokine	Hepatitis C Melanoma
Interferon β	Antiviral cytokine	Multiple sclerosis
Actimmune	Interferon γ	Chronic granulomatous disease (CGD), Osteopetrosis
Neupogen	G-CSF (hematopoietic cytokine)	Stimulates production of neutrophils Reduction of infection in cancer patients treated with chemotherapy
Leukine	GM-CSF (hematopoietic cytokine)	Stimulates production of myeloid cells after bone-marrow transplantation
Neumega	Interleukin 11 (IL-11), a hematopoietic cytokine	Stimulates production of platelets
Epogen	Erythropoietin (hematopoietic cytokine)	Stimulates red-blood cell production

Cytokines in Hematopoiesis

In Australia and Israel early studies demonstrated that soluble factors could support the growth and differentiation of red and white blood cells. The first of these soluble factors to be characterized, erythropoietin, was isolated from the urine of anemic patients and shown to support the development of red blood cells. Subsequently, many cytokines have been shown to play essential roles in hematopoiesis. During hematopoiesis, cytokines act as developmental signals that direct commitment of progenitor cells into and through particular lineages. A myeloid progenitor in the presence erythropoietin would proceed down a pathway that leads to the production of erythrocytes, suitable concentrations of a group of cytokines including IL-3, GM-CSF, IL-1, and IL-6 will cause it to enter differentiation pathways that lead to the generation of monocytes, neutrophils, and other leukocytes of the myeloid group.

Table 4.2. Haemopoietic cytokines used in clinical therapeutics

Hematopoietic growth factor	Sites of production	Main functions
Erythropoietin	Kidney, liver	Erythrocyte production
G-CSF	Endothelial cells, fibroblasts macrophages	Neutrophil production
Thrombopoietin	Liver, kidney	Platelet production
M-CSF	Fibroblasts, endothelial cells, macrophages	Macrophage and osteoclast production
SCF/c-*kit* ligand	Bone marrow stromal cells, constitutively	Stem cell, progenitor cells survival/division; mast cell differentiation
Flt-3 ligand	Fibroblasts, endothelial cells	Early progenitor cell expansion; pre-B cells
GM-CSF	T cells (TH1 and TH2), Macrophages, mast cells	Macrophage, granulocyte production; dendritic cell maturation and activation
IL-3	T cells (TH1 and TH2), macrophages	Stem cells and myeloid progenitor cell growth; mast cells
IL-5	Activated helper T cells –TH2 response only	Eosinophil production murine B-cell growth
IL-6	Activated T cells monocytes, fibroblasts endothelial cells	Progenitor cell stimulation; platelet production; immunoglobulin production in B cells
IL-11	Same as IL-6	
IL-7		T-cell survival

The participation of leukocytes in immune responses often results in their death and removal. However, both adaptive and innate immune responses generate cytokines that stimulate and support the production of leukocytes. A number of cytokines participate in hematopoiesis as Hematopoietic cytokines and a variety of cytokines are involved in supporting the growth and directing the differentiation of hematopoietic cells. Some additional factors may be required for some of the developmental pathways, e.g., CFU = colony-forming unit, a cell capable of generating a colony of cells from which the fully differentiated cell type emerges.

Cytokine Related Diseases

Defects in the complex regulatory networks governing the expression of cytokines and cytokine receptors have been implicated in a number of diseases, some of which are discussed as under:

Bacterial Septic Shock

Bacterial septic shock apparently develops because bacterial cell wall endotoxins stimulate macrophages to overproduce IL-1 and TNF-α to levels that cause septic shock. A study showed that injection of a recombinant IL-1 receptor antagonist (IL-1Ra), which prevents binding of IL-1 to the IL-1 receptor, resulted in a threefold reduction in mortality.

Lymphoid and Myeloid Cancers

Abnormalities in the production of cytokines or their receptors have been associated with some types of cancer. For example, abnormally high levels of IL-6 are secreted by cardiac myxoma cells, a benign heart tumour myeloma, plasmacytoma cells and cervical and bladder cancer cells. In myeloma cells, IL-6 appears to operate in an autocrine manner to stimulate cell proliferation. When monoclonal antibodies to IL-6 are added to in-vitro cultures of myeloma cells, their growth is inhibited. In addition, transgenic mice that express high levels of IL-6 have been found to exhibit a massive, fatal plasma cell proliferation, called plasmacytosis. Although these plasma cells are not malignant, the high rate of plasma cell proliferation possibly contributes to the development of cancer.

CONCLUSION

- Infectious agents can cause recurrent or persistent disease by avoiding normal host defense mechanisms or by subverting them to promote their own replication.
- There are many different ways of evading or subverting the immune responses.
- Antigenic variation, latency, resistance to immune effector mechanisms, and suppression of the immune response all contribute to persistent and medically important infections. In some cases, the immune response is part of the problem, some pathogens use immune activation to spread infection; others would not cause disease if it were not for the immune response. Each of these mechanisms teaches us something about the nature of the immune response and its weaknesses, and each requires a different medical approach to prevent or to treat infection.
- Infection with the human immunodeficiency virus (HIV) is the cause of acquired immune deficiency syndrome (AIDS).
- This worldwide epidemic is now spreading at an alarming rate, especially through heterosexual contact in less-developed countries.
- HIV is an enveloped retrovirus that replicates in cells of the immune system. Viral entry requires the presence of CD4 and a particular chemokine receptor, and the viral cycle is dependent on transcription factors found in activated T cells.
- Infection with HIV causes a loss of CD4 T-cells and an acute viremia that rapidly subsides as cytotoxic T-cell responses develop, but HIV infection is not eliminated by this immune response.
- HIV establishes a state of persistent infection in which the virus is continually replicating in newly infected cells.
- The current treatment consists of combinations of viral protease inhibitors together with nucleoside analogues and causes a rapid decrease in virus levels and a slower increase in CD4 T-cell counts.

- The main effect of HIV infection is the destruction of CD4 T-cells, which occurs through the direct cytopathic effects of HIV infection and through killing by CD8 cytotoxic T cells. As the CD4 T-cell counts wane, the body becomes progressively more susceptible to opportunistic infection with intracellular microbes.
- Eventually, most HIV-infected individuals develop AIDS and die; however a small minority (3 7%), remain healthy for many years, with no apparent ill effects of infection.
- The existence of such people and other people who have been naturally immunized against infection gives hope that it will be possible to develop effective vaccines against HIV. Whereas most infections elicit protective immunity, most successful pathogens have developed some means of evading a fully effective immune response, and some result in serious, persistent disease.
- In addition, some individuals have inherited deficiencies in different components of the immune system, making them highly susceptible to certain classes of infectious agent.
- Persistent infection and immunodeficiency illustrate the importance of innate and adaptive immunity in effective host defense against infection and present huge challenges for future immunological research.
- The human immunodeficiency virus (HIV) combines the characteristics of a persistent infectious agent with the ability to create immunodeficiency in its human host, a combination that is usually slowly lethal to the patient.
- The key to fighting new pathogens like HIV is to develop our understanding of the basic properties of the immune system and its role in combating infection more fully.
- Allergic reactions are the result of the production of specific IgE antibody to common, innocuous antigens.
- Allergens are small antigens that commonly provoke an IgE antibody response. Such antigens normally enter the body at very low doses by diffusion across mucosal surfaces and therefore trigger a TH2 response.

- The differentiation of naive allergen-specific T-cells into TH2 cells is also favored by the presence of an early burst of IL-4, which seems to be derived from a specialized subset of T-cells.
- Allergen-specific TH2 cells produce IL-4 and IL-13, which drive allergen-specific B-cells to produce IgE. The specific IgE produced in response to the allergen binds to the high affinity receptor for IgE on mast cells, basophils, and activated eosinophils.
- IgE production can be amplified by these cells because, upon activation, they produce IL-4 and CD40 ligand. The tendency to IgE over-production is influenced by genetic and environmental factors. Once IgE is produced in response to an allergen, re-exposure to the allergen triggers an allergic response.

FREQUENTLY ASKED QUESTIONS

Q1. What are cytokines? What role do they play in the immune system?

Answer: Cytokines are a diverse group of non-antibody proteins that act as mediators between cells. They play a main role in the natural or innate response by means of the direct action of mechanisms against the invading agent during the early stages of the infection, or by means of immune-modulatory mechanisms which activate NK cells and monocytes-macrophages; which then induce the release of cytokines.

Q2. Describe in brief the various types of cytokines.

Answer: Cytokines are bioactive hormones, normally glycoproteins, which exercise a wide variety of biological effects on those cells which express the appropriate receptors. Cytokines are designated by their cellular origin such that Monokines include those interleukins produced by macrophages/ monocytes, lymphokines include those interleukins produced by lymphocytes and Interleukins is used for cytokines which mostly influence cellular interactions. All cytokines are cyto-regulatory proteins with molecular weights under 60 kDa (in most cases under 25 kDa). They are produced locally, have very short half-lives (a matter of seconds to minutes), and are effective at picomolar concentrations. The effects of cytokines may be paracrine (acting on cells near the production locus), or autocrine (the same cell both produces, and reacts to, the cytokine).

Q3. What are chemokines?

Answer: Chemokines are a family of Chemoattractant cytokines (small proteins secreted by cells that influence the immune system) which play a vital role in cell migration through venules from blood into tissue and vice versa, and in the induction of cell movement in response to a chemical (chemokine) gradient by a process known as chemotaxis. In addition, chemokines also regulate lymphoid organ development and T-cell differentiation, mediate tumour cell metastasis, and have recently been shown to have a function in the nervous system as neuromodulator.

Q4. What is the difference between a chemokine and a cytokine?

Answer: Cytokines are signalling molecules produced by cell for specific biological functions. For example, interleukin is a type of cytokine produced by white cells as signalling molecules. Chemokine is a type of cytokine that is produced as a "chemo-attractant molecules" i.e., to attract cells to sites of infection/inflammation e.g., Interleukin 8. Cytokine is a general term used for all signalling molecules while chemokines are specific cytokines that functions by attracting cells to sites of infection/inflammation.

Q5. What Do Structures Tell Us About Chemokine Receptor Function?

Ans. Chemokine receptor structures with small molecules reveal the complicated and diverse structural foundations of small molecule antagonism and allostery, and highlight the inherent physicochemical challenges of receptor: chemokine Sinterfaces. The structures promote unique an understanding of chemokine receptor biology.

Q6. What are the various types of chemokines?

Answer: Chemokines are grouped and named according to their amino acid composition, particularly on the first two cysteine residues of a conserved tetra-cysteine motif. The CC and CXC chemokines form the two largest groups. The molecules CX3CL1, XCL1 and XCL2 are also regarded as chemokines. There are forty-seven known chemokines and nineteen chemokine receptors, and this numerosity results in a high degree of specificity. In fact, the particular molecules expressed on a cell determine which tissue a cell will migrate into. For example, cells expressing the chemokine receptor CCR7 migrate to lymph nodes, where their ligands, CCL19 and CCL21, are expressed. Chemokines may also be grouped according to their function, such as whether they are inflammatory or homeostatic. Inflammatory chemokines are produced when inflamed tissue releases cytokines such as tumour necrosis factor (TNF), and they function to recruit leukocytes. Homeostatic chemokines are expressed constitutively and play a key role in lymphocyte migration to, and the development of, lymphoid organs. Furthermore the CXC chemokines can be grouped as to whether they are angiogenic or angiostatic. The CXC chemokines containing the ELR amino acid motif (CXCL1-3, 5-8, 14 and 15) tend to be angiogenic, whereas ELR negative CXC chemokines are mainly angiostatic, with CXCL12 being a possible exception.

Q7. What are the benefits of using cytokines as immune modulators?

Answer: Cytokines play a key role in modulation of immune responses. Cytokine networks regulate lymphocyte turnover, differentiation, and activation. Many different cell types, in addition to immune cells, produce cytokines and express receptors for cytokines. Cell-to-cell communication (cellular "crosstalk") is maintained via cytokine networks. In disease, these networks undergo imbalance. By measuring amplification or down regulation of cytokine signalling cascades in response to pathological insults or therapeutic interventions, it might be possible to evaluate disease progression or regression.

MULTIPLE CHOICE QUESTIONS

Q1. Therapy for immediate hypersensitivity includes injection of antigen (allergen) to …

A. Induce wheal and flare.
B. Increase T-cells making IL-4.
C. Cause anaphylaxis.
D. Increase T cells making IFNγ.

Q2. Cell-mediated immune responses are …

A. Enhanced by depletion of complement.
B. Suppressed by cortisone.
C. Enhanced by depletion of T cells.
D. Suppressed by antihistamine.
E. Enhanced by depletion of macrophages.

Q3. Mast cell products mediate some of the symptoms of immediate hypersensitivity by increasing …

A. IgE receptors.
B. Secretion of IgE.
C. Capillary leakage.
D. Secretion of IgG.

Q4. Immediate hypersensitivity usually involves …

A. Mast cells.
B. Antibodies to mast cells.
C. Platelets.
D. IgG.

Q5. NK cells are more numerous during …

A. Early secretory phase of the menstrual cycle.
B. Late secretory phase of the menstrual cycle.
C. Early proliferative phase of the menstrual cycle.
D. Late proliferative phase of the menstrual cycle.

Q6. Control of the activated complement components results from ...

A. Agglutination.

B. Immune adherence.

C. Instability and inactivation of some of these components.

D. Mobility of phagocytes.

Q7. All of the following are true about acute phase proteins EXCEPT ...

A. They include C-reactive protein.

B. They include complement proteins.

C. They are mainly produced in the liver.

D. They function to limit tissue damage.

E. They are not induced by cytokines.

Q8. Complement inhabitory proteins include the following EXCEPT ...

A. Decay accelerating factor (DAF).

B. CD59 (protectin).

C. Membrane cofactor protein (MCP).

D. ICAM-1.

Q9. B cells are distinguished from T cells by the presence of ...

A. CD3.

B. CD4.

C. CD8.

D. Surface Ig.

E. Class I MHC antigen.

Q10. Lymphocytes of the mucosal immune system ...

A. Are normally primed in the lamina propria of the intestine.

B. Home mainly to mucosal sites and not systemic lymphoid organs.

C. Make up less than 10% of the lymphoid tissues in the body.

D. Mainly produce IgG antibodies.

E. Are only of the T cell type.

Q11. Newborns …

A. Receive IgM antibodies from the mother through placental transfer.
B. Have virtually a full complement of maternal IgG antibodies.
C. Have very few lymphocytes in their circulation.
D. Respond to antigens as well as adults.
E. Receive maternal B cells.

Q12. Rearrangement of VH genes begins during …

A. The pre-B cell stage.
B. The pro-B cell stage.
C. Maturation of B cells into plasma cells.
D. Development of dendritic cells.
E. Thymus development.

Q13. All of the following are true about the development of blood cells EXCEPT …

A. cytokines are required
B. IL-7 is involved in T cell development.
C. M-CSF is required for granulocyte development.
D. B cell development takes place mainly in the bone-marrow.

Q14. Allotypes are …

A. Antigenic determinants which segregate within a species.
B. Critical to the function of the antibody combining site.
C. Involved in specificity.
D. Involved in memory.

Q15. IgE …

A. Is bound together by J chain.
B. Binds to mast cells through its Fab region.
C. Differs from IgG antibody because of its different H chains.
D. Is present in high concentration in serum.

Answer Key

1 (D), 2 (B), 3 (C), 4 (A), 5 (B), 6(C), 7(E), 8(D), 9(D), 10(B), 11(B), 12(B), 13(C), 14(A), 15(C).

ASSIGNMENTS

Q1. What do you understand by therapeutic cytokines?
Q2. Explain role of cytokines in immune response.
Q3. How do cytokines work as an immune therapy?
Q4. What role do cytokines play in inflammatory disorders?
Q5. Explain cytokine therapy for treating malignancies.

REFERENCES

Asadullah K, Sterry W, Volk HD. 2003. Interleukin-10 therapy—review of a new approach. *Pharmacol. Rev.* 55:241–269.

Bosio CM, Bielefeldt-Ohmann H, Belisle JT. 2007. Active suppression of the pulmonary immune response by Francisella tularensis Schu4. *J. Immunol.* 178:4538–4547.

Cameron CE, Castro C. 2001. The mechanism of action of ribavirin: lethal mutagenesis of RNA virus genomes mediated by the viral RNA-dependent RNA polymerase. *Curr. Opin. Infect. Dis.* 14:757–764.

Casadevall A. 1996. Antibody-based therapies for emerging infectious diseases. *Emerg. Infect. Dis.* 2:200–208.

Chacko AM, Li C, Pryma DA, Brem S, Coukos G, Muzykantov V. Targeted delivery of antibody-based therapeutic and imaging agents to CNS tumors: crossing the blood-brain barrier divide [published correction appears in Expert Opin Drug Deliv. 2013 Oct;10(10):1463]. *Expert Opin Drug Deliv.* 2013;10(7):907–926.

Cheng XW, Lu JA, Wu CL, Yi LN, Xie X, Shi XD, Fang SS, Zan H, Kung HF, He ML. 2011. Three fatal cases of pandemic 2009 influenza A virus infection in Shenzhen are associated with cytokine storm. *Respir. Physiol. Neurobiol.* 175:185–187.

Chung F. 2001. Anti-inflammatory cytokines in asthma and allergy: interleukin-10, interleukin-12, interferon-gamma. *Mediators Inflamm.* 10:51–59.

Coates ARM, Hu Y. 2007. Novel approaches to developing new antibiotics for bacterial infections. *Br. J. Pharmacol.* 152:1147–1154.

Conlan JW, Zhao XG, Harris G, Shen H, Bolanowski M, Rietz C, Sjostedt A, Chen WX. 2008. Molecular immunology of experimental primary tularemia in mice infected by respiratory or intradermal routes with type A Francisella tularensis. *Mol. Immunol.* 45:2962–2969.

Dambuza IM, He C, Choi JK, et al. IL-12p35 induces expansion of IL-10 and IL-35-expressing regulatory B cells and ameliorates autoimmune disease. *Nat Commun*. 2017;8(1):719.

de Castro IF, Guzman-Fulgencio M, Garcia-Alvarez M, Resino S. 2010. First evidence of a pro-inflammatory response to severe infection with influenza virus H1N1. *Crit. Care* 14:115.

D'Elia RV, Harrison K, Oyston PC, Lukaszewski RA, Clark GC. Targeting the "cytokine storm" for therapeutic benefit. *Clin Vaccine Immunol.* 2013;20(3):319–327.

Descotes J. Immunotoxicity of monoclonal antibodies. *MAbs.* 2009;1(2):104–111. doi:10.4161/mabs.1.2.7909.

Finlay BB, McFadden G. 2006. Anti-immunology: evasion of the host immune system by bacterial and viral pathogens. *Cell* 124:767–782.

Fischbach MA, Walsh CT. 2009. Antibiotics for emerging pathogens. *Science* 325:1089–1093.

Fleming A. 1929. On the antibacterial action of cultures of a penicillium, with special reference to their use in the isolation of B. influenzae. *Br. J. Exp. Pathol.* 10:226–236.

Fujio K, Okamura T, Sumitomo S, Yamamoto K. Therapeutic potential of regulatory cytokines that target B cells. *Int Immunol.* 2016;28(4):189–195.

Ganança L, Oquendo MA, Tyrka AR, Cisneros-Trujillo S, Mann JJ, Sublette ME. The role of cytokines in the pathophysiology of suicidal behavior. *Psychoneuroendocrinology*. 2016;63:296–310.

Kutateladze M, Adamia R. 2010. Bacteriophages as potential new therapeutics to replace or supplement antibiotics. *Trends Biotechnol.* 28:591–595.

Lee S, Margolin K. Cytokines in cancer immunotherapy. *Cancers (Basel)*. 2011;3(4):3856–3893.

Mares CA, Ojeda SS, Morris EG, Li Q, Teale JM. 2008. Initial delay in the immune response to Francisella tularensis is followed by hypercytokinemia characteristic of severe sepsis and correlating with upregulation and release of damage-associated molecular patterns. *Infect. Immun*. 76:3001–3010.

Moreno H, Gallego I, Sevilla N, de la Torre JC, Domingo E, Martin V. 2011. Ribavirin can be mutagenic for arenaviruses. *J. Virol.* 85:7246–7255.

Opal SM, Depalo VA. 2000. Anti-inflammatory cytokines. *Chest* 117:1162–1172.

Oyston PCF, Sjostedt A, Titball RW. 2004. Tularaemia: bioterrorism defence renews interest in Francisella tularensis. *Nat. Rev. Microbiol.* 2:967–978.

Parker WB. 2005. Metabolism and antiviral activity of ribavirin. *Virus Res.* 107:165–171.

Piret J, Boivin G. 2011. Resistance of herpes simplex viruses to nucleoside analogues: mechanisms, prevalence, and management. Antimicrob. *Agents Chemother.* 55:459–472.

Parisi L, Toffoli A, Ghiacci G, Macaluso GM. Tailoring the Interface of Biomaterials to Design Effective Scaffolds. *J Funct Biomater.* 2018;9(3):50.

Perrone LA, Plowden JK, Garcia-Sastre A, Katz JM, Tumpey TM. 2008. H5N1 and 1918 pandemic influenza virus infection results in early and excessive infiltration of macrophages and neutrophils in the lungs of mice. *PLoS Pathog.* 4:e1000115.

Radfar L, Ahmadabadi RE, Masood F, Scofield RH. Biological therapy and dentistry: a review paper. *Oral Surg Oral Med Oral Pathol Oral Radiol*. 2015;120(5):594–601.

Rose-John S, Heinrich PC. Soluble receptors for cytokines and growth factors: generation and biological function. *Biochem J*. 1994;300:281–90.

Sachdeva N, Asthana D. Cytokine quantitation: technologies and applications. *Front Biosci*. 2007;12:4682–95.

Sharma J, Mares CA, Li Q, Morris EG, Teale JM. 2011. Features of sepsis caused by pulmonary infection with Francisella tularensis type A strain. *Microb. Pathog*. 51:39–47.

Shenoi S, Friedland G. 2009. Extensively drug-resistant tuberculosis: a new face to an old pathogen. *Annu. Rev. Med.* 60:307–320.

Sun L, He C, Nair L, Yeung J, Egwuagu CE. Interleukin 12 (IL-12) family cytokines: Role in immune pathogenesis and treatment of CNS autoimmune disease. *Cytokine*. 2015;75(2):249–255.

Tisoncik JR, Korth MJ, Simmons CP, Farrar J, Martin TR, Katze MG. 2012. Into the eye of the cytokine storm. *Microbiol. Mol. Biol.* Rev. 76:16–32.

Udwadia ZF. 2012. Totally drug-resistant tuberculosis in India: Who let the djinn out? *Respirology* 17:741–742.

Us D. 2008. Cytokine storm in avian influenza. *Mikrobiyol. Bul.* 42:365–380.

Van den Bergh JMJ, Smits ELJM, Versteven M, et al. Characterization of Interleukin-15-Transpresenting Dendritic Cells for Clinical Use. *J Immunol Res*. 2017;2017:1975902.

Wang SY, Le TQ, Kurihara N, Chida J, Cisse Y, Yano M, Kido H. 2010. Influenza virus-cytokine-protease cycle in the pathogenesis of vascular hyperpermeability in severe influenza. *J. Infect. Dis.* 202:991–1001.

Whiteside TL. Assays for cytokines. In: Thompson AW, Lotze MT, editors. *Cytokine Handbook*. 4. Amsterdam: Academic Press; 2003. pp. 1375–96. 6 plates.

In: Cytokines and Their Therapeutic Potential ISBN: 978-1-53617-017-7
Editor: Manzoor Ahmad Mir

Chapter 5

CHEMOKINES AND CYTOKINES IN INFECTIOUS DISEASES

Nissar A. Wani, Umar Mehraj, Safura Nisar, Bashir Ahmad Sheikh, Syed Suhail Hamdani, Hina Qayoom and Manzoor Ahmad Mir*

Department of Bioresources, School of Biological Sciences, University of Kashmir, Srinagar Jammu and Kashmir, India

ABSTRACT

Recent developments in the understanding of cytokine biology and the importance of such compounds in regulating inflammatory and other immune responses have led to a wave of studies in examining the role of these mediators in disease processes. While playing a pivotal role in host defense against infection, cytokines also contribute to pathology when released in excessive amounts. Much work, both in academic institutions and in the biotechnology and pharmaceutical industries, has been done to the development of cytokine or anti-cytokine treatment strategies in infectious diseases. Although some strategies have failed, but there have been numerous successes that have led to effective interventions for

---

* Corresponding Author's Email: drmanzoor@kashmiruniversity.ac.in.

inflammatory and infectious diseases. As research advances and tools are improved to understand the immune system, more is being learned about cytokines. There is an increased interest in harnessing the language of the immune system to direct its responses and improve health. This research holds great potential, though the road to its realization will likely be riddled with failed experiments and confounding results. Cytokine therapy is not merely a tool for the future, years from the grasp of our medical science cabinets. To its contrary, several cytokine therapies are now routinely available and used by many people living with a number of infectious diseases including HIV.

Keywords: anti-microbial, therapeutics, bioterrorism, globalisation, infectious diseases, cytokines, chemokines, anti-cytokine, biotechnology, chemoattractant, neuromodulator, toxic, sputum, macrophages, antibodies, therapies, allergy, psoriasis, atherosclerosis, malaria, phagocytosis, leucocytes

OBJECTIVES

- Overview of cytokines and chemokines.
- To have a basic understanding about chemokines.
- Discuss about cytokines and their types.
- Role of cytokines and chemokines in infectious diseases.
- Describe applications of cytokines/chemokines in immunotherapy.

INTRODUCTION

Cytokines are signalling proteins, usually less than 80 kDa in size (usually 5-20kDa), which regulate a wide range of biological functions including innate and acquired immunity, haematopoiesis, inflammation, repair and proliferation mostly through extracellular signalling. They are secreted by many cell types and are involved in cell-to-cell interactions, and they predominantly function in a paracrine fashion. They may also act at a distance by secretion of soluble products into the circulation i.e., endocrine or systemic effect and may have effects on the cell itself as autocrine effect. Cytokines exist in broad families that are structurally related but exhibit diverse function e.g., the TNF/TNF receptor super family, interleukin IL-1 super family, and IL-6 super family. Cytokines can act as: Mediators of the innate immunity like: inflammation, Chemotaxis, activation of macrophage and NK cells. They also play a role in adaptive immunity both humoral and cellular (Figure 5.1). Cytokines also act as regulators of lymphocyte activation, proliferation and differentiation. They can also act as stimulators of the growth of hematopoietic stem cells.

Types of Cytokines

Each cytokine has a matching cell-surface receptor. Subsequent cascades of intracellular signalling then alter cell functions. This may include the up regulation i.e., increased expression and/or down regulation i.e., decreased expression of several genes and their transcription factors resulting in the production of other cytokines. An increase in the number of surface receptors for other molecules, or the suppression of their own effects by feedback inhibition. The receptors for many cytokines have been grouped into super families' based on the presence of common homology regions. The various types of cytokines include:

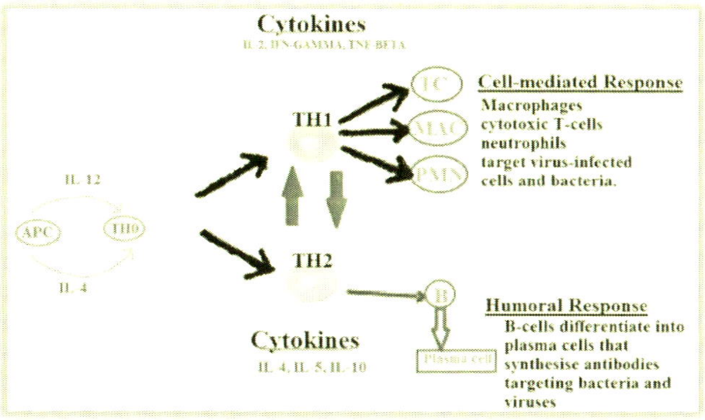

Figure 5.1. Cytokines are mediators of both humoral and cell-mediated immune responses.

Interleukins

Interleukins are a class of cytokines primarily expressed by leukocytes. They are glycoproteins involved in the signalling of many types of immune system functions. There are 17 different families of interleukins. Some of the more important ones include inflammatory mediators such as IL-1, IL-4, and IL-6, the potent anti-inflammatory IL-10, and other interleukins involved with T and B-cell signalling, following antigen presentation.

Interferons

Interferons are protein cytokines that have antiviral functions. They can activate macrophages and natural killer (NK) cells to attack and lyse virus-infected cells. One common interferon is IFN-gamma, a pyrogen involved in inflammatory response and macrophage as well as NK cell activation. IFN-gamma is produced by T-cells, both CD4 and CD8 and NK cells.

Tumour Necrosis Factor

Tumour necrosis factor (TNF) is a cytokine that induce apoptosis in abnormal cells such as tumour cells. It is a protein released by NK cells, macrophages and helper T-cells, typically in systemic immune responses. TNF-α is the most notable example. This long-lasting inflammatory mediator and pyrogen can cause fever and inflammation for up to 24 hours. It also stimulates acute phase reaction in the liver, a component of systemic immune system activation where the liver makes proteins involved in immune system response such as complement proteins. TNF-α is released in very high amounts in response to lipopolysaccharide i.e., infection with gram negative bacteria, which facilitates much of the self-destructive immune response in septic shock. In these cases, TNF-α, can cause organ failure from tissue hypo-perfusion, caused by damage and blood clotting from an overactive immune response.

Chemokines

Chemokines are a type of cytokine i.e., a short-lived secretory protein that regulates the function of nearby cells and may be described more specifically as chemotactic cytokines, because of their ability to cause certain cells in close proximity to undergo directed chemotaxis i.e., cellular movement in response to chemical signals. Cells that respond to chemokines migrate along a chemical signal gradient that is marked by increasing chemokine concentration, such that the cells end up in areas with comparatively high chemokine levels. In this way, chemokines that are secreted by cells at sites of inflammation attract immune cells to those sites, thereby aiding the immune response. Their actions are mediated by a family of 7-transmembrane G-protein–coupled receptors, the size of which have grown considerably in recent years and now include 18 members. Chemokine receptor expression on different cell types and their binding and response to specific chemokines are highly variable. Chemokine receptors have recently been implicated in several disease states including allergy, psoriasis, atherosclerosis, and malaria (Figure 5.2). However, most fascinating has been the observation that some of these receptors are used by human immunodeficiency virus type 1 in gaining entry into permissive cells.

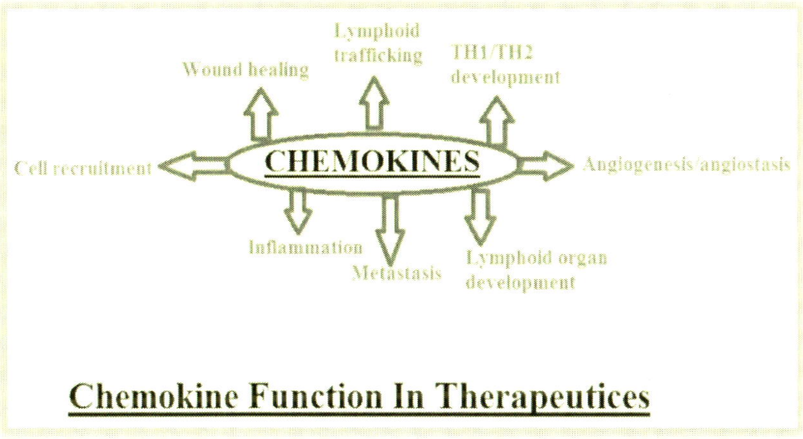

Figure 5.2. Chemokine function in clinical therapeutics.

Phagocytic leukocytes of the immune system undergo rapid and directed movements in chemo attractant gradients, a property that enables them to serve as the first line of cell-mediated host defense against infection. The interaction of chemo attractants with leukocytes initiates a series of coordinated biochemical and cellular events that includes alterations in ion fluxes, integrin avidity and transmembrane potential, changes in cell shape, secretion of lysosomal enzymes, production of superoxide anions, and enhanced locomotion. Two groups of chemo attractants have been identified and extensively studied. The "classical" chemo attractants, such as bacterial-derived N-formyl peptides, complement fragment peptides C5a and C3a, and lipid molecules such as leukotriene-B4 and platelet-activating factor. Recently, a number of chemotactic cytokines in the 8- to 17-KD molecular mass range have been shown to be selective chemo attractants for leukocyte sub-populations in-vitro and to elicit the accumulation of inflammatory cells in-vivo. These chemotactic cytokines belong to the chemokine super family,

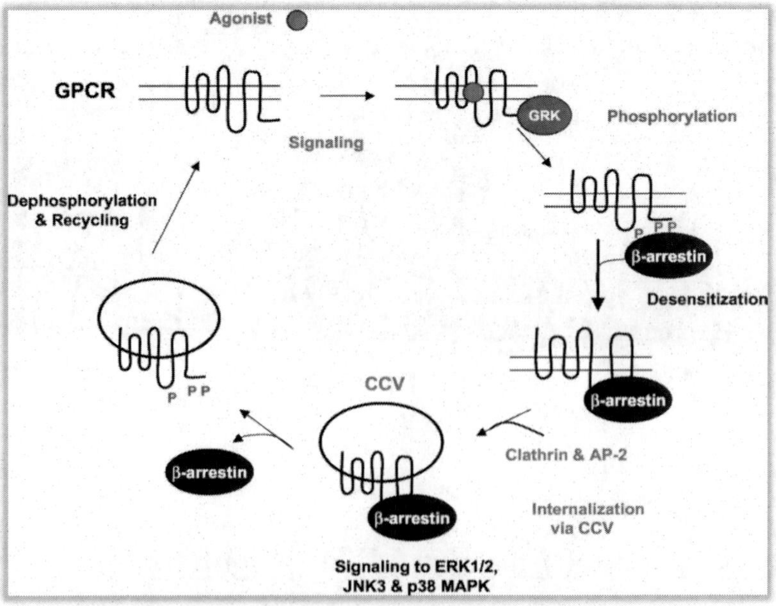

Figure 5.3. Cytokine receptors in a number of signaling processes.

which can be divided into 4 groups as: CXC, CX3C, CC, and C according to the positioning of the first 2 closely paired and highly conserved cysteines of the amino acid sequence. The specific effects of chemokines on their target cells are mediated by members of a family of 7-transmembrane–

spanning, G-protein–coupled receptors. These chemokine receptors are part of a much bigger super family of G-protein–coupled receptors that include receptors for hormones, neurotransmitters, paracrine substances, inflammatory mediators, certain proteinase, taste and odorant molecules, and even photons and calcium ions (Figure 5.3).

Chemokine Receptors in Inflammation

Leukocyte activation in acute inflammation: To reach sites of inflammation or injury, circulating leukocytes must exit the bloodstream by traversing the endothelium. Leukocytes usually attach to the apical surface of the endothelium of post-capillary venules, where the shear stress is lowest. The first step in the process of leukocyte recruitment at sites of inflammation is the generation of transient selectin-mediated interactions that cause tethering and rolling of flowing leukocytes on the endothelial cell surface. The slow velocity of rolling leukocytes on selectins favours encounters with chemokines that are presented on the apical surface of the endothelium by glycos-aminoglycans (GAGs). Chemokines bind to their respective chemokine receptors expressed on the leukocyte cell surface, leading to the alteration of β2 integrin avidity, especially CD11b/CD18, on the leukocyte cell surface. Then β2 integrin bind to their Ig counter-ligands, such as ICAM-1, ICAM-2, and ICAM-3, which have been up-regulated on the endothelial cell surface by pro-inflammatory cytokines. These interactions provide firm attachment of leukocytes to the endothelium and facilitate leukocyte haptotactictransendothelial migration. The binding of chemokines to their respective leukocyte receptors also initiates a series of cellular events, all of which aim to eradicate the infiltrating inflammatory agents. These events include changes in cell shape leading to enhanced locomotion, secretion of lysosomal enzymes, and production of superoxide anions. Once leukocytes reach the source of inflammation, a cytokine-rich milieu is generated that is sustained until the invading antigen is eliminated. In general, immune responses do not produce endothelial injury; however, on occasion acute or chronic inflammation may occur in which the endothelium and surrounding tissues become damaged, for example, by neutrophil-generated products.

Inflammation Resolution and Inflammatory Disorders

After acute infection or injury, blood vessels may be damaged. Part of the mechanism of wound healing, the formation of new blood vessels, known as angiogenesis, is a process tightly regulated by numerous biologic mediators, among them chemokines: CXC chemokines, such as IL-8, GRO-α, GRO-β, PF-4, IP-10, and Mig, have been implicated in the regulation of keratinocytes and endothelial cell function, including the stimulation and inhibition of proliferation, angiogenesis, angiostasis, and cell migration. However, evidence concerning the expression of chemokine receptors by endothelial cells has been conflicting. Recent data now shows that endothelial and epithelial cells express several functional chemokine receptors, in particular CXCR4. It has been proposed that endothelial proteoglycans can present chemokines to leukocyte and to endothelial-expressed chemokine receptors. This model is analogous to the way in which basic fibroblast growth factor is thought to bind to endothelial proteoglycans, facilitating its interaction with high-affinity fibroblast growth factor receptors on the endothelial cell surface. A low level of expression and responsiveness of chemokine receptors on endothelial cells may be sufficient to permit cell activation in the presence of high levels of proteoglycan-bound chemokine on the adjacent endothelial cell surface. These findings suggest that chemokines and their receptors may play an important role in the vascular remodelling and maintenance associated with inflammatory resolution.

Role of Cytokines in Immune Responses

Cytokines are involved in a staggeringly broad array of biological activities including innate immunity, adaptive immunity, inflammation and haematopoiesis. The main cytokines that have a role in the innate responses are: IL-1, IL-6, IL-12, IL-16, TNF α, INF α and β. The IL-1, IL-6 and IL-12 activate the monocytes-macrophages and NK cells (Fig 5.4). Tumour necrosis factor is the main trigger of the inflammatory response. TH cells exert most of their helper functions through secreted cytokines. Although CTLs also secrete cytokines, their array of cytokines generally is more restricted than that of TH cells. Antigen stimulation of TH cells in the presence of certain cytokines can lead to the generation of subpopulations of helper T-cells known as TH1 and TH2. Each subset displays characteristic and different profiles of cytokine secretion. The main cytokines that have a role in adaptive immune response are: IL-2, IL-4, IL-5, TGF β, IFN γ.

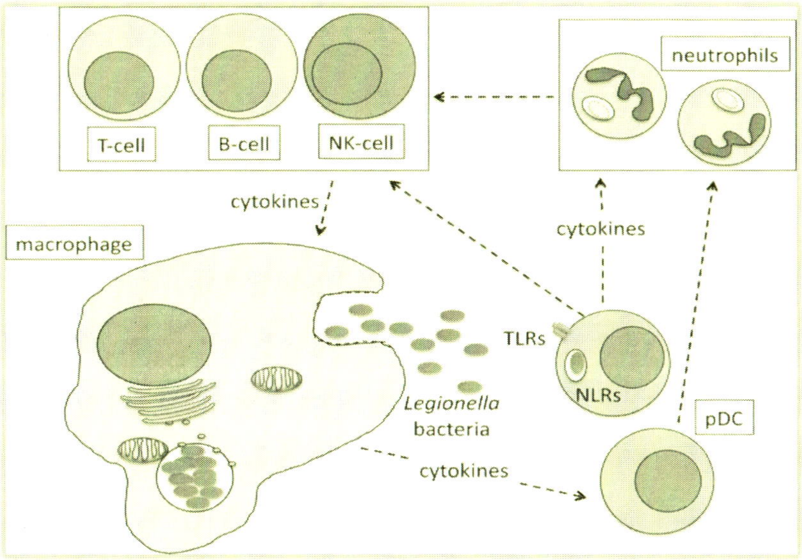

Figure 5.4. Role of cytokines in various immune responses.

A number of cytokines induce innate immune responses, because they include macrophage and NK-cell activation, developing an inflammatory and chemotaxis process. The cytokines having role in the innate response are: IL-1, IL-6, IL-12, TNF-α, IFN-α and β. The IL-1, IL-6, IL-12 activate the monocytes-macrophages and NK-cells. Tumor necrosis factor (TNF) is the main trigger of inflammatory response.

Table 5.1. List of cytokines involved in innate immune response

Cytokine	Synthesized by	Effects
IL-1	Monocytes, macrophages, epithelial cells and endothelial cells.	Inflammation, fever, induction of acute phase proteins.
IL-6	Macrophages, endothelial cells and T_H2 cells.	Influences adaptive immunity, induction of acute phase proteins.
IL-12	Macrophages, dendritic cells.	NK-cells, influences adaptive immunity.
TNF-α	Macrophages, monocytes, neutrophils, activated T-cells and NK-cells.	Inflammation, induction of acute phase proteins, neutrophil activation.
IFN-α	Macrophages, dendritic cells, virus-infected cells.	Activates NK-cells, increases class I MHC expression.
IFN-β	Macrophages, dendritic cells, virus-infected cells.	Activates NK-cells, increases class I MHC expression.

Table 5.2. List of cytokines involved in adaptive immune responses both humoral and cell-mediated immune response

Cytokine	Synthesized by	Effects
IL-2	T-cells.	T-cell proliferation, NK cell activation and proliferation, B-cell proliferation.
IL-4	Mast cells, T_H2 cells.	Promotes T_H2 differentiation, isotype switch to IgE.
IL-5	T_H2 cells.	Eosinophil activation and generation.
TGF-β	T-cells, macrophages, other cell types.	Inhabits T-cell proliferation and B-cell proliferation, promotes isotype switching to IgA.
IFN-γ	T_H1 cells, $CD8^+$ cells, NK-cells.	Activates macrophages, increases expression of class I and II MHC, increases antigen presentation.

Cytokines are also involved in the development and regulation of both cellular and humoral adaptive immune responses. T helper cells exert most of their helper functions through secreted cytokines. The main cytokines that have a role in adaptive immune responses are: IL-2, IL-4, IL-5, TGF-β, and IFN-γ.

Cytokines and Disease

Bronchial Asthma

Bronchial asthma is an inflammatory disease of the airways and is associated with bronchial hyper reactivity and reversible airway obstruction. Studies indicate that T-cell derived cytokine production rather than eosinophil influx or IgE synthesis is usually related to altered airway behaviour. There is an increase in the number of CD4+ helper T-cells in the airways which are predominantly of the TH2 subtype. TH2 cells are characterized by secretion of IL-4, IL-5, IL-9 and IL-13. Increased expression of pro-inflammatory cytokine TNF-α enhances the inflammatory process and has been linked to disease severity. IL-4 is the key cytokine in asthma and is involved in TH2 cell differentiation and IgE production. It stimulates the mucus producing cells and fibroblasts implicating its role in the pathogenesis of airway remodelling. In atopic asthmatics, IL-4 induces airway eosinophilia and causes bronchial hyper responsiveness. IL-5 is the primary cytokine involved in the production, differentiation, maturation and activation of eosinophils. It is crucial for inducing eosinophil infiltration in the airways. IL-13 is present in increased amounts in asthmatic airways and has very similar biological activities to IL-4. IL-4 induces IgE dependent mast cell activation involved in immediate type allergic/hypersensitivity reactions. In the asthmatic lung, IL-4 promotes cellular inflammation by induction of vascular cell adhesion molecule (VCAM-1) on the vascular endothelium.

Pleiotropic Activities of Th2 Cytokines in Allergic Asthma

When a naive T-cell encounters an antigen in presence of antigen presenting cells like macrophages, dendritic cells etc, they induce the secretion of type 2 T-helper cells. These activated type 2 T-helper cells influence the production of cytokines like IL-4, IL-5, IL-9 and IL-13. Among these cytokines IL-4, IL-9 and IL-13 binds to B-lymphocytes stimulating the expression of IgE antibodies. Further, these IgE antibodies bind to high affinity IgE receptor i.e., FcεRI on target mast cells. This high affinity IgE receptor activates sphingosine kinase dependent calcium mobilization in mast cells leading to degranulation with the release of inflammatory mediators like histamine, prostaglandin D2 and leukotriene which in turn acts on smooth muscle cells to induce bronchoconstriction. On the other hand, IL-5 and IL-9 act on eosinophils causing their activation, maturation and differentiation and finally leads to tissue damage.

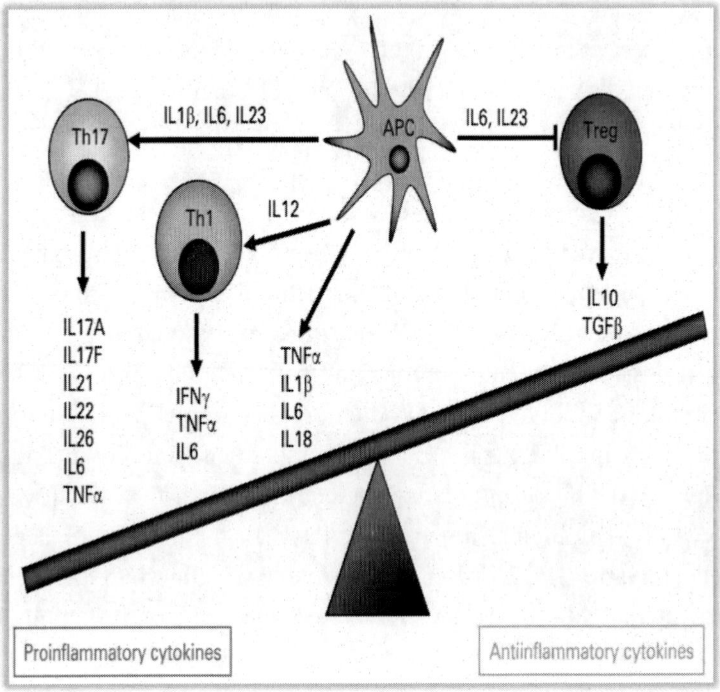

Figure 5.5. Action of pro-inflammatory and anti-inflammatory cytokines in immune responses.

Chronic Obstructive Pulmonary Disease

Cytokines released predominantly from T cells orchestrate the inflammation. Increased expression of IL-4 occurs in BAL fluid from patients with COPD. IL-4 is crucial for differentiation of TH2 cells from TH0 cells and may be important in initial sensitization to allergens. IFN-γ is the predominant cytokine in inflammation in patients and it orchestrates the infiltration of TH1 and Tc cells in the lungs through up-regulation of chemokine receptor CXCR3 on these cells and with the release of CXCR3 activating chemokines like CCL9, CCL10 and CCL11. Increased expression of IL-18 occurs in the alveolar macrophages in the airways of COPD patients and has been linked to disease severity. Sputum and BAL fluid express increased amount of pro-inflammatory cytokines TNF-α, IL-1 and IL-6 (Figure 5.5). Elevated levels of chemokines like CCL2 also appear in sputum, BAL fluid and lungs of COPD patients and are also expressed by alveolar macrophages, T-cells and epithelial cells.

HIV Infection

HIV infection results in deregulation of the cytokine profile both in vitro and in vivo. An important role is played by cytokines in controlling the homeostasis of the immune system. Secretion of TH1 cytokines such as IL-2 and IFN-γ is decreased while production of TH2 cytokines IL-4, IL-10 and pro inflammatory cytokine like IL-1, IL-6, IL-8 and TNF-α is increased at the time of HIV infection. Further, TNF-α, TNF-β, IL-1 and IL-6 stimulate HIV replication in T-cells and monocyte derived macrophages (MDM). So this type of an abnormal cytokine production impairs the cell mediated immunity thus contributing to the pathogenesis of the disease. IL-2, IL-7 and IL-5 up-regulates HIV-1 in T-cells while macrophage colony stimulating factor (M-CSF) stimulates HIV in MDM. IFN-α, IFN-, and IL-16 are HIV suppressive cytokines which inhibit HIV-1 replication in T-cells and MDM whereas, IL-10 and IL-13 inhibits it in MDM only. IFN-γ, IL-4 and GM-CSF, which are bi-functional cytokines, have shown both inhibitory and stimulatory effects for HIV infection.

Cytokines and Immunotherapy

Advances in the understanding of the role of cytokines in immune and inflammatory disorders have led to the development of cytokine-based therapies. Therapies have been developed with the express aim to block/inhibit or restore the activity of specific cytokines. Cytokines delivered by gene therapy and antisense oligonucleotide treatment are also being assessed. Currently, the most utilized approach to cytokine therapy is that of blocking or neutralizing cytokine action with monoclonal antibodies (mAbs). Drugs that block inflammatory cytokines, such as tumour necrosis factor, TNF-α are among the most successful therapeutics approved for clinical use.

Cytokine Immunotherapy

Immunotherapy is a medical term defined as the "treatment of disease by inducing, enhancing, or suppressing an immune response." The active agents of immunotherapy are collectively called immune modulators. They are a diverse array of recombinant, synthetic and natural preparations, often cytokines, such as granulocyte colony-stimulating factor (G-CSF), interferons, imiquimod and cellular membrane fractions from bacteria are already licensed for use in patients. Others including IL-2, IL-7, and IL-12, various chemokines, synthetic cytosine phosphate-guanosine (CpG), oligodeoxynucleotides and glucans are currently being investigated extensively in clinical and preclinical studies. The field of cytokines came of age in the late 1970s with the introduction of molecular biological approaches that resulted first in the cloning of IFNs, initially IFN-β by Tada Taniguchi and IFN-α by both Charles Weissman's group and David Goeddel's colleagues. By the mid-1980s, there was a plethora of well-defined cytokines and cytokine receptors that could be unambiguously studied, using molecular tools, such as cDNA probes, and antibodies that had been produced to recognize the pure recombinant proteins. All this was a long way from the 1960s and 1970s, when all researchers had were many uncharacterized bioactivities in cell supernatants termed simply by activity, e.g., lymphocyte-activating factor, macrophage-activating factor, and leukocyte pyrogen. All the tools available by the mid-1980s enabled researchers to assess the expression of cytokines in physiologic and pathologic states. The up regulated expression of cytokines in many different disease states led to an investigation of their role in the pathogenesis of disease. As cytokines are potent rate-limiting extracellular molecules, they are excellent targets for the products of the biotechnology industry, namely monoclonal antibodies and antibody-like receptor: Fc fusion proteins. These form the most specific therapeutics, more specific than small molecule organic chemicals, due to the greater surface of interaction of receptors and antibodies with their targets.

Cytokines in Immune and Inflammatory Disorders

Cytokines mediate a wide variety of biological activities that are relevant to autoimmune diseases, including inflammation induced by an immune response, as well as tissue repair and remodelling. The roles of different cytokines in autoimmune diseases have been widely studied. It has become clear that excessive production of pro inflammatory cytokines, as well as the relative paucity of regulatory cytokines contribute to the immune pathogenesis of these diseases. Restoring optimal cytokine balance may have therapeutic value that theoretically could be achieved either by blocking inflammatory cytokines or inducing or providing anti-inflammatory ones. To date, approved cytokine therapy in clinical practice is limited to the use of interferons. Rheumatoid arthritis is a common autoimmune disease, with approximately 1% prevalence in the industrialized world, and cytokine expression in this disease has been extensively analysed, an effort helped considerably by the accessibility of the diseased tissue. The first big success of anti-cytokine therapy, in the form of TNF-α blockade, was demonstrated in this disease, and it has now been repeatedly shown that blocking this single cytokine has marked beneficial effects on all aspects of disease activity and can prevent further joint destruction. In addition, it has been determined that several other important chronic diseases respond to TNF-α blockade. Due to the ease of performing clinical trials with well-established protocols, multiple cytokine blockade clinical trials have been performed in severe RA. These clinical trials have had variable success, and it is not understood why in this disease, as in many others, there are differences between results in animal models, where many anti-cytokine therapies are very effective, and the human disease, treatment of which is proving more challenging.

Multiple sclerosis (MS) is an important neurodegenerative disease in which inflammation and cytokines are prominent in the affected tissue. In multiple sclerosis (MS) activated auto-reactive T-cells, B-cells, and other mononuclear cells cross the blood–brain barrier and enter the central nervous system (CNS). These mononuclear cell infiltrates, together with resident CNS cells, can cause injury to oligodendrocytes and myelin. There are at least four clinical subtypes of this disease. The relapsing-remitting form is the most common (80–85%) and is characterized by acute attacks (relapses) followed by remissions. Failure to recover from relapse is a major cause of disability but up to 30–50% of these patients accrue additional disability with subclinical relapses (secondary progressive phase MS). Human beta interferon (IFN-β) has been demonstrated to modulate many of these processes. Two forms of IFN-β are in clinical use: IFN-β1a and IFN-β1b. Despite some differences in their pharmacologic properties they have similar clinical effects. Seven large, randomized placebo-controlled trials have demonstrated clinical efficacy in both relapsing-remitting (three studies) MS and secondary progressive (four studies) MS. These trials have consistently demonstrated that both forms of IFN-β reduce disease activity by reducing clinical attack rate and magnetic resonance imaging (MRI) activity measures. IFN-β treatment seems also to improve disease severity in MS; however these data are less convincing. The more recent clinical studies have focused on the impact of dose and optimal dosing frequency. The currently available data suggest that higher dose and/or more frequent administration may increase the efficacy of IFN-β treatment in MS.

Cytokines as cure for infectious diseases remains an ever-growing health concern worldwide due to increasing antibiotic-resistant microbial strains, immune-compromised populations, international traffic and globalisation, and bioterrorism. There exists an urgent need to develop novel prophylactic and therapeutic strategies. In addition to classic antibiotic therapeutics, immune-modulatory molecules such as cytokines or their inhibitors represent a promising form of antimicrobial therapeutics or immune adjuvant used for the purpose of vaccination. These molecules, in the form of either recombinant protein or transgene, exert their antimicrobial effect by enhancing infectious agent-specific immune activation or memory development, or by dampening undesired inflammatory and immune responses resulting from infection and host defence mechanisms. In the last two decades, a number of cytokine therapy-based experimental and clinical trials have been conducted, and some of these efforts have led to the routine clinical use of cytokines. For instance, although IFNs have been used to treat hepatitis C with great success, many other cytokines are yet to be fully evaluated for their antimicrobial potential.

CONCLUSION

- Cytokines and chemokines are an important class of effector molecules that play a fundamental role in orchestrating the innate and acquired immune responses needed to eliminate or war off invading pathogens.
- In recent years, its being witnessed that an outpouring of information on the role of cytokines and chemokines in human infectious diseases.
- These studies have led to a deeper understanding of the pathogenesis of infectious diseases.
- While playing a pivotal role in host defence against infection, cytokines also contribute to pathology when released in excessive amounts.
- Cytokines also play a role in the pathogenesis of sepsis and septic shock.
- Cytokine and anti-cytokine-based therapies have already entered the mainstream of medical practice.
- Regulatory agencies continue to approve anti-cytokine therapies for patients with rheumatoid arthritis, and it appears that many more cytokines will be approved in the near future for treatment of diseases.
- There has been rapid recent progress in the understanding of the biology of chemokines and their receptors. This progress has seen

an increase in the association between chemokine receptors and certain human disease states.

Frequently Asked Questions

Q1. Does cytokine therapy lead to toxicity?

Answer: Therapy with cytokines often leads to dose-dependent side effects. Being pleiotropic in nature, cytokines are able to influence more than a single cell. Because of their short half-life, for better therapeutic effects it requires high doses, which may cause pleiotropic activities and ultimately lead to adverse effects. Administration of high dose of IL-2 for cancer immunotherapy stimulates the cytotoxic CD8+ T-cells and NK cells proliferation, which promotes tumour regression in the patients and leads to adverse reactions.

Q2. What do you understand by chemokine receptors?

Answer: In order for a cell to respond to a chemokine it must express a complementary chemokine receptor. Chemokine receptors belong to the vast family of G-protein coupled receptors (GPCRs): seven transmembrane receptors which bind extracellular ligands and consequently initiate intracellular signalling. When a chemokine binds its receptor a calcium signalling cascade is created, resulting in the activation of small GTPases. This then has downstream effects such as activation of integrins (molecules involved in cell adhesion) and actin polymerisation, resulting in the development of a pseudopodia (cellular projection), polarised cell morphology and ultimately cell movement.

Q3. What role do cytokines play in lymphocyte homeostasis?

Answer: The size of lymphocyte populations is regulated by replication and death. Cytokines produced by non-lymphoid cells provide key survival and replication signals for several lymphocyte subpopulations. The availability of these cytokines serves as a homeostatic regulatory mechanism by determining the upper limit of the population size. IL-7 is required for survival of naive CD4+ and CD8+ cells and memory CD8+ cells. IL-15 is required for survival of memory CD8+ cells. IL-12 and IL-4 also promote memory CD8+ survival BAFF is required for survival of mature B cells. Antigen receptor signals, together with these cytokine signals, are required for survival of mature B cells and naive T cells.

Q4. What is a cytokine storm?

Answer: Inflammation is the body's first line of defense against infection or injury, responding to challenges by activating innate and adaptive responses. Throughout its activation, the inflammatory response must be regulated to prevent a damaging systemic inflammation, also known as a "cytokine storm" in the host which can result in significant pathology and ultimately death. A number of cytokines with anti-inflammatory properties are responsible for this, such as IL-10 and transforming growth factor β (TGF-β). Each cytokine acts on a different part of the inflammatory response. For example, products of the Th2 immune response suppresses the Th1 immune response and vice versa. Without the ability to resolve the inflammation, the collateral damage to surrounding cells has the potential to be catastrophic, resulting in sepsis and even death.

Q5. How do cytokines contribute to inflammatory mechanisms?

Answer: There are both pro-inflammatory cytokines and anti-inflammatory cytokines. Interleukin-1 (IL-1) and tumour necrosis factor (TNF), play a key role in orchestrating the mechanisms responsible for inflammation. These two cytokines induce production by many cells of lipid mediators, proteases, and free radicals, all of which play a direct role in development of the deleterious effects of inflammation. IL-1 and/or TNF exert cytotoxic effects on the vascular endothelium, cartilage, bone, muscle, or pancreatic beta-cell islets. Cytokines, including interferon gamma (IFN), IL-3 and granulocyte-macrophage colony-stimulating factor (GM-CSF), amplify the inflammatory response by increasing production of IL-1 and TNF by macrophages. Macrophages also produce other cytokines, such as IL-8 and macrophage Chemoattractant protein-1 (MCP-1), with Chemoattractant properties that contribute to draw leucocytes to the site of inflammation. IL-6, produced in large amounts during inflammatory processes, induces the production of acute phase proteins by hepatocytes. IL-1, TNF, IL-11, leukemia inhibitory factor (LIF), and transforming growth factor beta (TGF beta) share this effect. TGF beta also has a number of anti-inflammatory effects. TGF beta, IL-4, and IL-10 inhibit production of IL-1 and TNF. Glucocorticoids also have this effect. Glucocorticoids can be produced as a result of a chain of events initiated by IL-1, TNF, and IL-6 and involving the neuro-endocrine axis. Other substances, such as IL-1 receptor antagonist (IL-1 ra) or soluble forms of the TNF receptors can specifically inhibit the effects of IL-1 and TNF. Cascade production of cytokines, inhibition, negative feed-back, and synergistic mechanisms are parameters that illustrate the concept of "cytokine network" and aptly characterize the role of these mediators in the mechanisms of inflammation.

Q6. What are interleukins?

Answer: Interleukins are a subset of a larger group of cellular messenger molecules called cytokines, which are modulators of cellular behaviour. Like other cytokines, interleukins are not stored within cells but are instead secreted rapidly, and briefly, in response to a stimulus, such as an infectious agent.

Q7. What are interferons?

Answer: Interferons (IFNs) are a group of soluble glycoproteins that are produced and released from cells in response to virus infection (and other stimuli). They were first described in the late 1950s by two scientists – Isaacs and Lindenmann–who assigned an antiviral factor the name ‘interferon’. This was due to the molecule’s ability to ‘interfere’ with the growth of the influenza virus.

MULTIPLE CHOICE QUESTIONS

Q1. Which among the following is true about Interleukin-4 (IL-4)

A. Activates B-cells, switching them to produce IgE (allergies)
B. Activates strong cell mediated responses
C. Activates T-cells, causing proliferation
D. Activates vascular endothelium and increases vascular permeability

Q2. Tumour necrosis factor-α (TNF-α) is:

A. Is a cell signalling protein involved in systemic inflammation?
B. Activates T-cells, causing proliferation
C. Activates vascular endothelium and increases vascular permeability
D. Differentiates CD4 cells

Q3. TH1 cells are:

A. Follicular dendritic cells, surrounded by B-cells and T-cells to trigger immune response
B. Langerhans or inter-digitating cells
C. produce interferon-gamma, interleukin (IL)-2, and tumour necrosis factor (TNF)-beta
D. Produces antibody responses and regulates B-cells

Q4. Hormonal systems are commonly characterized by feedback inhibition. In contrast to hormones, many cytokines amplify responses by up-regulation of their own receptors on target cells. An example of this mechanism is seen in which of the following?

A. The differential cytokine expression of TH1 and TH2 cells.
B. The chemokine concentration gradient resulting in chemotaxis.
C. The stimulation of CD4+ T cells by IL-2.
D. The effect of cytokines on osteoblastic differentiation.

Q5. A patient presents with a bacterial infection characterized by fever. This fever is due to which of the following?

A. Proliferation of the bacteria.

B. Antibody responses to the bacteria.

C. Bacterial infection of the hypothalamus.

D. Cytokines produced by phagocytes.

Q6. Following a skin abrasion and local minor infection, scar tissue is normally formed. This is due to proliferation of fibroblasts and deposition of extracellular material and is stimulated by which of the following?

A. Granulocyte-colony stimulating factor (G-CSF).

B. IL-1.

C. TGF-β.

D. IL-17.

Q7. Which among following is true about Interleukin-γ (IL- γ):

A. Activates B-cells, switching them to produce IgE (allergies)

B. Activates strong cell mediated responses

C. Activates T-cells, causing proliferation

D. is primarily secreted by activated T cells and natural killer (NK) cells

Q8. Patients suffering from toxic shock syndrome are found to have which of the following as the causative mechanism?

A. High levels of bacterial toxins.

B. Excessive levels of bacterial-specific antibodies.

C. Generation of bacterial-specific cytotoxic T cells.

D. Massive stimulation of helper T cells irrespective of antigenic specificity.

Q9. The signature cytokines produced by th1 cells

A. IL-10

B. IFN-γ and sometimes IL-2

C. TNF-A

D. IL-6

Q10. Patients with Hodgkin's lymphoma frequently have eosinophils associated with the malignant cells in the lymph nodes and eosinophilia (high eosinophil levels) in their blood. This is due to the increased production of which cytokine by the malignant cells?

A. IL-1.

B. IL-10.

C. TNF-α.

D. IL-5.

Q11. Cytokines primarily involved in T cell proliferation and developments are

A. IL-2 and IL-7

B. IL-12

C. IL-4 and IL-5

D. TNF-β

Q12. Which of the following statements regarding the functional properties of cytokines is false?

A. They typically have pleiotropic properties.

B. They often exhibit functional redundancy.

C. They often display antigen specificity.

D. They exhibit synergistic or antagonistic properties.

Q13. All of the following are induced by the chemokine IL-8 except

A. Activation of neutrophils.

D. Wound healing.

C. Extravasation of neutrophils.

D. Reduction of cytokine production by T H cells.

Q14. Which of the following cytokines plays a role in terminating inflammatory responses?

A. IL-2

B. IL-4

C. TGF-b

D. IFN-a

Q15. Cytokines always act

A. By binding to specific receptors.

B. Always in an autocrine fashion.

C. At long range.

D. Antagonistically with other cytokines.

Answer Key

1(C), 2(A), 3(C), 4(C), 5(D), 6(C), 7(D), 8(D), 9(B), 10(D), 11(A), 12(C), 13(D), 14(C), 15(A).

Assignments

Q1. What do you understand by cytokine based therapy?

Q2. What is immunotherapy and how does it help in treating diseases?

Q3. What role do chemokines play in HIV?

Q4. What role do cytokines play in rheumatoid arthritis?

Q5. How do chemokines work?

References

Ao X., Stenken J. A. Microdialysis sampling of cytokines. *Methods.* 2006;38:331–41.

Asadullah K., Sterry W., Volk H. D. 2003. Interleukin-10 therapy—review of a new approach. *Pharmacol. Rev.* 55:241–269.

Baggiolini M, Dewald B, Moser B. Human chemokines: an update. *Annu Rev Immunol.* 1997;15:675.

Baggiolini M, Dewald B, Moser B. Interleukin-8 and related chemotactic cytokines CXC and CC chemokines. *Adv Immunol.* 1994.

Chung F. 2001. Anti-inflammatory cytokines in asthma and allergy: interleukin-10, interleukin-12, interferon-gamma. *Mediators Inflamm.* 10:51–59.

de Castro I. F., Guzman-Fulgencio M., Garcia-Alvarez M., Resino S. 2010. First evidence of a pro-inflammatory response to severe infection with influenza virus H1N1. *Crit. Care* 14:115.

Elliott, M. J., et al. 1993. Treatment of rheumatoid arthritis with chimeric monoclonal antibodies to tumor necrosis factor alpha. *Arthritis Rheum.* 36:1681-1690.

Feldmann, M., Brennan, F. M., Maini, R. N. 1996. Role of cytokines in rheumatoid arthritis. *Annu. Rev. Immunol.* 14:397-440.

Feldmann, M., Maini, R. N. 2001. Anti-TNF alpha therapy of rheumatoid arthritis: what have we learned? *Annu. Rev. Immunol.* 19:163-196.

Finlay B. B., McFadden G. 2006. Anti-immunology: evasion of the host immune system by bacterial and viral pathogens. *Cell* 124:767–782.

Gerard C., Gerard N. P. C5A anaphylatoxin and its seven transmembrane-segment receptor. *Annu Rev Immunol.* 1994.

Goeddel, D. V., et al. 1980. Synthesis of human fibroblast interferon by E. coli. *Nucleic Acids.*

Goldman D. W., Goetzl E. J. Specific binding of leukotriene B4 to receptors on human polymorphonuclear leukocytes. *J Immunol.* 1982.

Hanahan D. J. Platelet activating factor: a biologically active phosphoglyceride. *Annu Rev Biochem.* 1986;55:483.

Hibbs (Jr.), J. B., Taintor, R. R., Chapman (Jr.), H. A., Weinberg, J. B. 1977. Macrophage tumor killing: influence of the local environment. *Science.* 197:279-282.

Masihi K. N. 2003. Progress on novel immunomodulatory agents for HIV-1 infection and other infectious diseases. *Expert Opin. Ther. Pat.* 13:867–882.

Murdoch C, Finn A. 2000. Chemokine receptors and their role in inflammation and infectious diseases. *Blood* 95:3032–3043.

Murphy P. M. The molecular biology of leukocyte chemoattractant receptors. *Annu Rev Immunol.* 1994;12:593.

Opal S. M., Depalo V. A. 2000. Anti-inflammatory cytokines. *Chest* 117:1162–1172.

Oppenheim, J. J. 2001. Cytokines: past, present, and future. *Int. J. Hematol.* 74:3-8.

Schiffmann E., Corcoran B. A., Wahl S. M. N-formylmethionyl peptides as chemoattractants for leucocytes. *Proc Natl Acad Sci U.S.A.* 1975;72:1059.

Signore A., Procaccini E., Annovazzi A., Chianelli M., van dLC, Mire-Sluis A. The developing role of cytokines for imaging inflammation and infection. *Cytokine*. 2000;12:1445–54.

Tisoncik J. R., Korth M. J., Simmons C. P., Farrar J., Martin T. R., Katze M. G. 2012. Into the eye of the cytokine storm. *Microbiol. Mol. Biol. Rev.* 76:16–32.

Tsou C. L., Gladue R. P., Carroll L. A., et al. Identification of C-C chemokine receptor 1 (CCR1) as the monocyte hemofiltrate C-C chemokine (HCC)-1 receptor. *J Exp Med.* 1998;188:603.

Vilcek, J., Feldmann, M. 2004. Historical review: cytokines as therapeutics and targets of therapeutics. *Trends Pharmacol. Sci.* 25:201-209.

GLOSSARY

Acquired immune deficiency syndrome (AIDS): A progressive immune deficiency caused by infection of CD4 T cells with the human retrovirus HIV.

Active immunity: usually long-lasting immunity that is acquired through the production of antibodies and memory T cells within the organism in response to the presence of antigens.

Adaptive immune system: also called the acquired immune system, this component of the immune system comprises white blood cells, particularly lymphocytes. When it is presented with a new microbe or vaccine, it may take days or weeks to respond or adapt, but the resultant improved immune readiness, or "memory," is sustained for long periods (years).

Adenosine deaminase (ADA): an enzyme found in mammalian tissues that are capable of catalyzing the process in which adenosine is split into inosine and ammonia. A deficiency can cause problems with metabolic reactions in cells, which leads to the destruction of B and T cells. ADA deficiency can lead to one form of severe combined immune-deficiency disease.

Allergy: Originally defined as altered reactivity on second contact with antigen; now usually refers to a type I hypersensitivity reaction.

Antibody: a protein on the surface of B cells that is also secreted in large amounts into the blood or lymph in response to an antigen, a component within an invader such as a bacterium, virus, parasite, or transplanted organ. Antibodies neutralize the antigen, and thereby the invader, by binding to it, often directing it toward a macrophage for destruction. Also called an immunoglobulin.

Antigen: a foreign substance (usually a protein or carbohydrate) capable

Antiretroviral drugs: drugs that act against retroviruses (such as HIV).

APCs (antigen-presenting cells): A variety of cell types that carry antigen in a form that can stimulate lymphocytes.

Apoptosis: Programmed cell death that involves nuclear fragmentation and condensation of cytoplasm, plasma membranes, and organelles into apoptotic bodies.

Arthus reaction: Inflammation seen in the skin some hours following injection of antigen. It is a manifestation of a type III hypersensitivity reaction.

Atopy: The clinical manifestation of type I hypersensitivity reactions, including eczema, asthma, rhinitis, and food allergy.

Autocrine: This refers to the ability of a cytokine to act on the cell that produced it.

Autoimmune disorders: conditions in which the body's own immune system acts against it.

Autoimmunity: Immune recognition and reaction against the individual's own tissue.

Auto reactive: describes immune cells that mount a response against the body's own cells or tissues.

B cell co-receptor complex: A group of cell surface molecules consisting of complement receptor type 2 (CD21), CD81, and CD19, which act as a co-stimulatory receptor on mature B cells.

B cells: Lymphocytes that develop in the bone marrow in adults and produce antibody. They can be subdivided into two groups, B1 and B2. B1 cells use minimally mutated receptors, which are close to the germline immunoglobulin sequences, whereas B2 cells are the major responding population in conventional immune responses to protein antigens.

Basophil: A population of polymorphonuclear leukocytes that stain with basic dyes and have important roles in the control of inflammation.

Biochemicals: chemicals produced within living organisms. Many coordinate to fight off invasion in an immune response.

Biological barriers: the body's first layer of protection against harmful microbes; skin is a prime example.

Blood-brain barrier: a tight layer of cells and tissue that separates the brain from the rest of the body; a physical roadblock that normally keeps immune cells outside the brain.

Blood-forming stem cells: immature cells in the bone marrow that multiply extensively and produce red and white blood cells and platelets.

CD4+ helper T cells: T cells with CD4 receptors that respond to antigens on the surface of specific molecules by secreting a certain type of cytokine that stimulates B cells and killer T cells. Helper T cells are infected and killed by HIV; people who develop AIDS have no more than one-fifth the normal number of helper T cells.

Central nervous system: the brain and spinal cord, to which sensory impulses are transmitted and from which motor impulses emanate. The central nervous system supervises and coordinates the activity of the entire nervous system and interacts with the immune system.

Chemokines: A large group of cytokines falling into four families, of which the main families are the CC and the CXC group. Chemokines are designated as ligands belonging to a particular family (e.g., CCL2). Many chemokines have older descriptive names, for example CCL2 is macrophage chemotactic protein-1 (MCP-1). They act on G protein linked, seven-transmembrane pass receptors and have a variety of chemotactic and cell-activating properties.

Chemo kinesis: Increased random migratory activity of cells.

Chemotaxis: Increased directional migration of cells, particularly in response to concentration gradients of certain chemotactic factors..

Clones: copies that viruses make of themselves.

Cytokine: a class of substance secreted by cells of the immune system to regulate immune cells.

Cytokines: A generic term for soluble molecules that mediate interactions between cells..

Cytotoxic T cells: Cells that can kill virally infected targets expressing antigenic peptides presented by MHC class I molecules.

Dendritic cell: an antigen-presenting immune cell that initiates the immune response by activating lymphocytes and stimulating the secretion of cytokines. Dendritic cells also prevent autoimmune reactions by instructing the T lymphocytes to be silent or tolerant to the body itself.

DNA (deoxyribonucleic acid): nucleic acid that carries the cell's genetic information and is capable of self-replication and the synthesis of RNA.

DNA vaccine: vaccines that often use "naked" DNA (DNA not associated with a cell or a virus) with instructions for making protective antigens. When injected, the DNA is taken in by other cells, which then produce protective antigens.

E. coli: a bacterium that is used in public health as an indicator of fecal pollution (as of water or food) and in medicine and genetics as a research organism. E. coli occurs in various strains that may live as harmless inhabitants of the human lower intestine or may produce a toxin causing intestinal illness.

Enzymes: complex proteins produced by living cells and that catalyze specific reactions from biochemicals.

Eosinophils: A population of polymorphonuclear granulocytes that stain with acidic dyes and are particularly involved in reactions against parasitic worms and in some hypersensitivity reactions.

Epidemic: an outbreak of disease that simultaneously affects an atypically large number of individuals within a population, community, or region.

Epithelioid cells: A population of activated mononuclear phagocytes present in granulomatous reactions.

Estrogen: a steroid hormone produced chiefly by the ovaries, responsible for promoting development and maintenance of female secondary sex characteristics. Estrogen may play a role in certain immune system diseases.

Genetic engineering: deliberate alteration of genetic material by intervention in genetic processes.

Granulocyte: a type of phagocyte with cytoplasm that contains grain like particles.

Highly active antiretroviral therapy (HAART): a treatment to combat AIDS using several antiretroviral drugs at the same time.

Histamine: a compound found in mammalian tissues that cause stretching of capillaries, contraction of smooth muscle, and stimulation of gastric acid secretions; released during allergic reactions.

HIV (human immunodeficiency virus): The causative agent of acquired immune deficiency syndrome (AIDS).

Immune deficiency diseases (IDDs): diseases that result when one or more parts of the immune system are missing or defective.

Immunoglobulin E (IgE): a class of antibodies that function in allergic reactions.

Immunosuppressive: describes a treatment that suppresses natural immune responses—for example, chemotherapy for cancer.

Inactivated vaccines: vaccines made by growing and purifying large numbers of the target organism in the laboratory and then killing them with heat, radiation, or chemicals. The immune system reacts to the dead microorganisms, producing immunity.

Inflammation: a build-up of fluid and cells that occurs as the immune system fights a hostile invader.

Innate immune system: component of the immune system that consists of a set of genetically encoded responses to pathogens and does not change or adapt during the lifetime of the organism. Innate immunity involves quickly mobilized defenses triggered by receptors that recognize a broad spectrum of microbes; in contrast to adaptive immunity, it does not acquire memory for an improved response during a second exposure to infection.

Interferons (IFNs): A group of molecules involved in signaling between cells of the immune system and in protection against viral infections.

Interferons: Interferons are cytokines produced by the cells of the immune system in response to viral infection and other stimuli.

Interleukins (IL-1–IL-22): A group of molecules involved in signaling between cells of the immune system.

.**Interleukins:** Interleukins are cytokines produced and secreted mainly by CD3+ and CD4+ T lymphocytes. Interleukins promote development and differentiation of natural killer cells, T and B lymphocytes and hematopoietic stem cells.

killer T cell: a type of lymphocyte that directly attacks and kills infected cells or other targets, including tumor cells and even one's own tissues. Killer cells are generated by the coordinated action of dendritic cells and CD4+ helper T cells.

knockout: term used in genetic engineering when a specific gene is deliberately removed in order to create an organism unable to carry out the functions the gene codes for; knockouts are used by immunologists to determine the functions of specific genes that encode immune proteins.

Latency: the state or period in which a virus has invaded a host but is not actively multiplying, and during which symptoms of the infection are not seen. "Microbial latency" means the microbe is not multiplying, as occurs in some cells in HIV infection, while "clinical latency" means that the patient does not have symptoms of disease even though the virus is multiplying and damaging the immune system. In HIV, clinical latency precedes the AIDS stage.

Lymph nodes: small, rounded structures in the lymphatic system that contain disease-fighting white blood cells, especially lymphocytes, and filter out harmful microbes and toxins. Lymph nodes may become enlarged when they are actively fighting infection.

Lymphocyte: a type of white blood cell involved in the human body's immune system, of which there are two broad categories, T cells and B cells. Lymphocytes are an integral part of the body's defenses because they are highly specific for antigens associated with microbes, tumor cells, transplants, allergies, and tissues attacked in autoimmune diseases. The immune system comprises clones of lymphocytes, each with a single specificity, and exposure to antigens leads to clonal expansion, the acquisition of helper and killer functions, and formation of immune memory.

Lysozyme: an enzyme in saliva and tears that destroys bacteria.

Macrophages: large phagocyte cells that remove harmful microbes from the body.

Major histocompatibility complex (MHC) molecules: a group of molecules that help the immune system distinguish between harmful and safe foreign substances in the body. Recent research suggests some classes of MHC molecules also play an essential role in brain function.

Mast cells: large cells, found in connective tissues that mediate allergic reactions. Mast cells play an important protective role in wound healing and defend against pathogens.

Memory B and T cells: B and T cells that remain in the body after the completion of an immune response to ward off future attacks by the same microbe. Memory is imparted by the increased size in the antigen-specific B or T cell clone, as well as improved function of individual cells within the clone.

Microglia: specialized immune cells, related to macrophages that protect the central nervous system.

Molecular mimicry: an occurrence in many autoimmune disorders in which a microbe carries antigens that resemble those on a particular organ, causing the immune system to attack the body.

Monoclonal antibodies: antibodies derived from a single cell and used against a specific antigen such as a cancer cell. Rituxan and Herceptin are monoclonal antibodies used in the treatment of lymphoma and breast cancer, respectively.

Mutation: a process in which a microbe or organism undergoes a permanent change in hereditary material. When viruses or bacteria mutate they are no longer recognized by the immune system and become resistant to previously administered vaccines and drugs.

Myelin: a white, fatty material that sheathes nerves and enhances the transmission of signals between the brain and the body. In multiple sclerosis, an autoimmune disorder, immune cells attack myelin, affecting the transmission of nerve signals.

Pandemic: an outbreak of disease occurring over a wide geographical area and affecting an exceptionally high proportion of the population.

Passive immunity: immunity acquired by the transfer of antibodies (as by injection of serum from an individual with active immunity).

Pathogen: a specific causative agent of disease, such as a bacterium or a virus.

Penicillin: a mixture of nontoxic antibiotics produced by mold and used regularly to treat harmful bacteria.

Phagocyte: a cell such as a white blood cell that engulfs and consumes foreign material, such as microorganisms.

Plasma cell: an antibody-producing lymphocyte derived from a B cell upon reaction with a specific antigen.

Protease: an enzyme that catalyzes the splitting of proteins into smaller molecules. To treat AIDS, scientists have designed drugs that interfere with protease made by the HIV virus, which is essential to its replication.

Reassortment: the constant state of flux and rearrangement seen in the genes of viruses.

Red blood cells: any of the haemoglobin-containing cells that carry oxygen to the tissues and are responsible for the red color of vertebrate blood.

Regulatory T cells (Treg cells): special T cells that regulate or suppress immune responses, preventing autoimmunity for example.

Replication: process by which an organism produces a copy of itself—for example, the way microbes reproduce.

Respiratory syncytial virus (RSV): a virus that forms masses, or syncytia, in tissue culture and that is responsible for severe respiratory diseases.

Retrovirus: a type of RNA virus (such as HIV) that reproduces by transcribing itself into DNA (using reverse transcriptase). The resultant DNA inserts itself into a cell's DNA and is reproduced by the cell.

Reverse transcriptase (RT): an enzyme that catalyzes the formation of DNA using RNA as a template.

RNA (ribonucleic acid): a group of molecules similar in structure to a single strand of DNA. The function of RNA is to carry the information from the DNA in the cell's nucleus into the body of the cell to assemble proteins.

Rotavirus: a retrovirus with a double-layer protein shell and a wheel-like appearance. Rotaviruses cause diarrhea, especially in infants.

Stem cell transplants: a kind of passive immune therapy that transfers cells instead of antibodies. Stem cells have the capacity to give rise to all elements of the immune system, such as many types of lymphocytes and phagocytes.

Steroids: a large family of chemical substances, comprising many hormones, body constituents, and drugs; they are often immunosuppressive.

Subunit vaccines: vaccines that contain only a part of the target microorganism.

Synapses: specialized junctions at which cells of the nervous system signal to one another and to non-neuronal cells, such as those of muscles and glands.

T cell: a type of lymphocyte that possesses highly specific cell-surface antigen receptors; types include CD4+ helper T cells, regulatory T cells, and killer T cells.

Thymus: A primary lymphoid organ in the thoracic cavity over the heart.

Tolerance: the capacity of the body to become less responsive to a substance or a physiological insult. Tolerance to components of the self prevents or suppresses autoimmunity.

Toxoid vaccine: an inactivated and weakened version of the disease-causing toxin a microbe produces; it is still capable of inducing the formation of antibodies when injected.

Transgenic technology: technology used to deliberately alter the genome of an organism by the transfer of a gene or genes from another species or breed.

Two-photon microscopy: an imaging technique using high-powered laser microscopes to examine immune response in the nervous system.

Vaccine: killed microorganisms, weakened living organisms, fully virulent living organisms, or subunit proteins of a microbe, administered to produce or artificially increase immunity to a particular disease.

Vector vaccines: vaccines made by inserting protective antigen genes into harmless bacteria or viruses (vectors). As the vectors multiply in the body, they expose the immune system to protective antigens, stimulating active immunity against the harmful organism.

White blood cells: any of the blood cells that are colorless, lack hemoglobin, and contain a nucleus. They include the lymphocytes, dendritic cells, monocytes, neutrophils, eosinophils, and basophils; also called leukocytes.

About the Editor

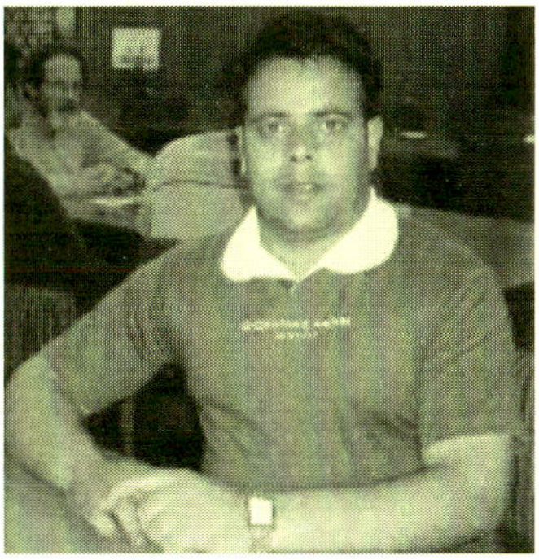

Dr. Manzoor Ahmad Mir, MSc, PhD, PGDHE, JRF-NET
Senior Assistant Professor
Coordinator/Head Department of Bioresources
School of Biological Sciences
University of Kashmir Srinagar-190006
E-mail ID: drmanzoor@kashmiruniversity.ac.in

Dr. Manzoor Ahmad Mir holds Master's Degree in Zoology from HNBG Central University after qualifying prestigious National level CSIR-JRF-NET examination and worked jointly for his Ph. D at Jawaharlal Nehru University New Delhi and CSIR-Institute of Microbial Technology Chandigarh in the field of Immunology and Cell Biology. He currently teaches Endocrinology, Animal Physiology, Immunology and Developmental Biology at the Department of Bioresources, University of Kashmir, and has been a Research Scientist at SATCAS Stroke Research Chair Majmaah University KSA. Dr. Manzoor has research and teaching experience of 13 years and has attended many courses and conferences on immunology, cancer Biology, stroke biology and endocrinology at USA, UK, Kuwait, China, UAE and Saudi Arabia. His basic research interests include molecular immunology, Tuberculosis immunology, Cancer and Stroke Biology. He has published more than 50 high-impact research papers and book chapters, in recognition of which he has received several awards and Royalties from international publishing houses. Dr. Manzoor has authored several books with international publishers like Elsevier USA and Nova Science Publisher USA. He is currently receiving Royalty from Academic Press USA for his book in the field of Immunology entitled "Developing costimulatory molecules for immunotherapy of diseases". Dr. Manzoor is on the editorial board of some prestigious journals from DOVE medical press New Zealand and Springer Plus UK and has been an invited speaker at various scientific meetings/conferences within India and abroad. He is member of many scientific organizations and societies like International Immunology Association, Indian Association of Immunology, Indian National Science Association, IMMUNOCON etc. Dr. Manzoor was awarded Teachers Associate Research Excellence Fellowship (TARE) by DST Govt of India. He has been awarded Summer Research Fellowship Programme (SRFP-2019) by Indian Academy of Sciences and National Science Academy. Dr. Manzoor has developed Massive Open Online Course (MOOCs) in Immunology for UG students by sanctioned by UGC-Consortium for Educational Communication (CEC) SWAYAM Ministry of HRD Govt of India. He has been awarded another MOOC Course on Endocrinology by Academic advisory committee of CEC-UGC.

About the Contributors

Dr. Nissar Ahmad Wani

Scientist D

Department of Biotechnology, School of Life Sciences

Central University of Kashmir, Ganderbal J&K India 191201

Email: waninh@yahoo.co.in

Mr. Umar Mehraj

Junior Research Fellow UGC-CSIR

Research Scholar

Department of Bioresources,

School of Biological Sciences,

University of Kashmir Srinagar-190006

E-mail: umarshk92@gmail.com

Miss Safura Nisar

Research Scholar

Department of Bioresources,

School of Biological Sciences,

University of Kashmir Srinagar-190006

E-mail: safooranisar99@gmail.com

Hina Qayoom
Research Scholar
Department of Bioresources,
School of Biological Sciences,
University of Kashmir Srinagar-190006
E-mail: hinaqkhan1@gmail.com

Bashir Ahmad Sheikh
Research Scholar
Department of Bioresources,
School of Biological Sciences,

Syed Suhail Hamdani
Research Scholar
Department of Bioresources,
School of Biological Sciences,
University of Kashmir Srinagar-190006
Email: sohailsyed.hamdani@gmail.com

INDEX

C

D

E

F

G

N

O

P

R

S

Related Nova Publications

Antiphospholipid Antibodies (APLA): Types and Functions in Health and Disease

Editor: Luke E. Ward

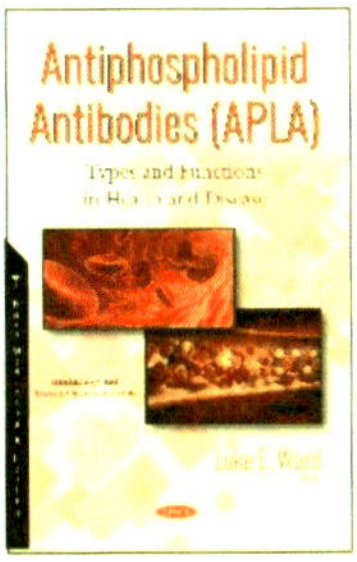

Series: Immunology and Immune System Disorders

Book Description: The opening chapter of *Antiphospholipid Antibodies (APLA): Types and Functions in Health and Disease* is focused on the modern immunoassays for the determination of aPL in biological fluids.

Softcover ISBN: 978-1-53613-971-6
Retail Price: $82

Old and Novel Humoral Biomarkers of Autoimmune Myasthenia Gravis

Authors: Giovanni Luca Masala, Davide G. Corda, M.D., Giovanni A. Deiana, Giannina Arru, and GianPietro Sechi, M.D.

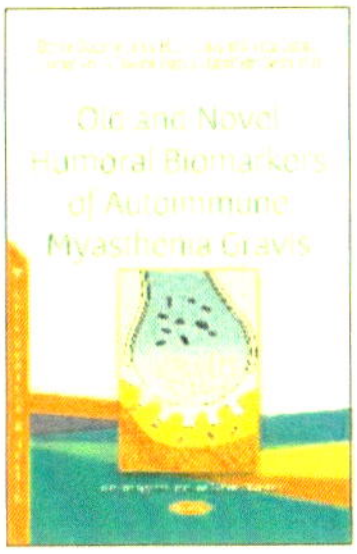

Series: Immunology and Immune System Disorders

Book Description: Autoimmune Myasthenia Gravis (MG) is mediated by pathogenic autoantibodies to components of the postsynaptic muscle endplate at the neuromuscular junction. Due to the clinical heterogeneity of the disease, there is a great need for objective biomarkers for diagnostic as well as therapeutic purposes.

Softcover ISBN: 978-1-53613-836-8
Retail Price: $95

To see a complete list of Nova publications, please visit our website at www.novapublishers.com

Related Nova Publications

Helper T Cells: Types, Functions and New Research

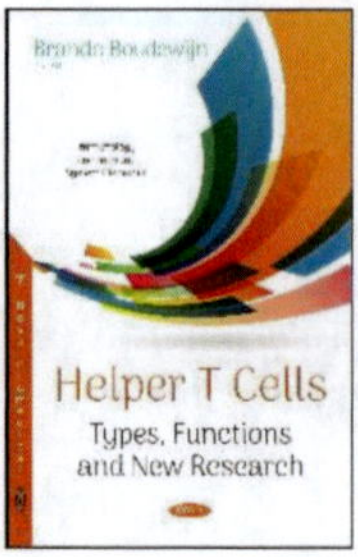

Editor: Brando Boudewijn

Series: Immunology and Immune System Disorders

Book Description: *Helper T Cells: Types, Functions and New Research* presents current research in the Tfh cell research field with a special focus on the maintenance of TFH cells and their fate once the immune response has resolved.

Softcover ISBN: 978-1-53613-070-6
Retail Price: $82

Chronic Granulomatous Disease: Genetics, Biology and Clinical Management

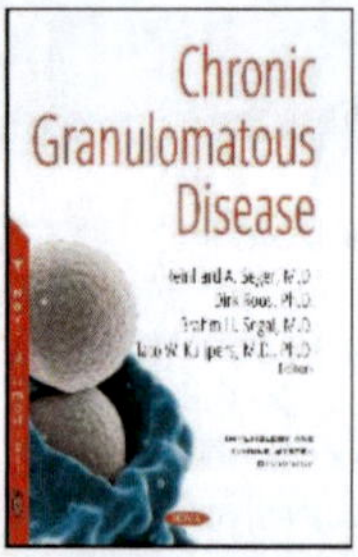

Authors: Reinhard A. Seger, Dirk Roos, Brahm H. Segal and Taco W. Kuijpers

Series: Immunology and Immune System Disorders

Book Description: This is the first e-book on Chronic Granulomatous Disease (CGD). This book is meant for everyone involved in the diagnosis, treatment or guidance of patients with this disease, as well as for the patients and their parents/caretakers, investigators and students experiencing this disease.

Online ISBN: 978-1-53612-498-9
Retail Price: $0

To see a complete list of Nova publications, please visit our website at www.novapublishers.com